Study Guide for Huber

Leadership and Nursing Care Management

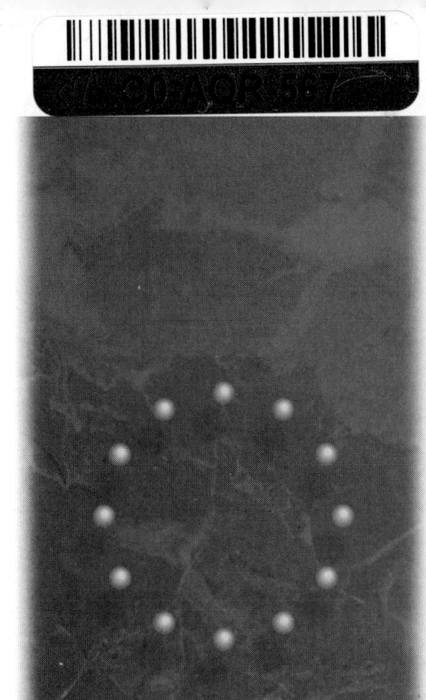

Second Edition

Jean Nagelkerk, RN, PhD, FNP-C
Professor and Director of Graduate Programs
Kirkhof School of Nursing
Grand Valley State University
Grand Rapids, Michigan

W.B. SAUNDERS COMPANY
A Harcourt Health Sciences Company
Philadelphia London Toronto Montreal Sydney Tokyo

W.B. SAUNDERS COMPANY
A Harcourt Health Sciences Company
The Curtis Center
Independence Square West
Philadelphia, PA 19106-3399

NOTICE

Nursing is an ever-changing field. Standard safety precautions must be followed, but as new research and clinical experience broaden our knowledge, changes in treatment and drug therapy become necessary or appropriate. Readers are advised to check the product information currently provided by the manufacturer of each drug to be administered to verify the recommended dose, the method and duration of administration, and the contraindications. It is the responsibility of the licensed prescriber, relying on experience and knowledge of the patient, to determine dosages and the best treatment for the patient. Neither the publisher nor the editor assumes any responsibility for any injury and/or damage to persons or property.

The Publisher

Study Guide for Huber
LEADERSHIP AND NURSING CARE MANAGEMENT ISBN 0-7216-9200-1

Printed in the United States of America

Last digit is the print number: 9 8 7 6 5 4 3 2 1

Contents

Answers to chapter-ending Study Questions in parent text supplied by

Linda D. Scott, PhD, RN
Assistant Professor of Nursing
Grand Valley State University
Grand Rapids, Michigan

Cynthia Arslanian-Engoren, PhD, RN, CNS
Assistant Professor
Madonna University
Livonia, Michigan

Overview of Nursing Administration

STUDY FOCUS

Health care is becoming increasingly complex, turbulent, and chaotic. Strong nurse administrators are needed who can manage complex health care systems through interdisciplinary collaboration. A nurse administrator combines clinical, administrative, financial, and operational skills to manage problems and provide high-quality, cost-effective health care in acute and primary settings. The two roles that nurses assume are direct care providers and care managers. Nurses are central to health care organizations and orchestrate continuity of care for clients. Nurses facilitate environmental factors, foster interdisciplinary collaboration, and distribute resources in providing direct care and case management to clients.

Nursing administration is very important in providing quality health care to communities. Nursing administration is the act of synthesizing management theory and nursing practice, using power and authority to provide quality care, and managing the health care delivery system to meet the community-based needs of clients. Nursing administration theory and knowledge is derived from three primary sources: nursing, management, and leadership theory. A systems view focuses on interrelationships among factors and goals, interdependencies, and transcends narrow discipline-specific views. Theory and concepts are also drawn from other sources such as anthropology, education, psychology, sociology, public health, business, and organizational management science. Integrating nursing knowledge and knowledge from a combination of disciplines enables nurses to gain new insights into clinical and administrative practice.

Nursing administration is complex and involves using three categories of nurses to provide quality health care to clients. *Nurse executives* provide leadership by developing strategic plans, implementing new programs, and coordinating the delivery of nursing services to clients. Nurse executives look at the "big picture" and make long-range decisions for the organization. *Nurse managers* help nurse executives by working on day-to-day management activities and coordinating nursing care at the unit level. *Nurse care providers* are integral to coordinating and providing direct care to clients. These categories of individuals work as a team to provide the best care possible.

All categories of nurses use leadership and management behaviors to accomplish their work. Leadership focuses on influencing people to accomplish goals, inspiring confidence, envisioning the future, and motivating followers by leading the way. Management, on the other hand, coordinates and integrates resources, plans, organizes, directs, controls, and accomplishes organizational goals. Leadership and management overlap by focusing on goal accomplishment and motivating and directing followers. The most effective nurses use both leadership and management behaviors to accomplish their goals and motivate other nurses and clients.

The nurse administrator's role is changing and requires skills in population-based care management across the lifespan. Evidence-based practice focuses on theory and research. The Iowa Model of Nursing Administration incorporates three levels of analyses, including patient aggregates, organizations, and health care. This model uses both systems and outcome perspectives to examine complexity in health care systems.

LEARNING TOOLS

Group Activity: Understanding Nursing Administration

Purpose: To help you understand how different disciplines enhance the practice of nursing, and to enable you to discuss the interdependence of nursing with other disciplines. The disciplines that will be explored are nursing, management, business, education, and psychology.

Divide the study group into five smaller groups.

Assign each group to either nursing, management, business, education, or psychology.

Each small group should take 20 minutes to identify material important for nursing administration. For example, one important item from business may be how to work with budgets. Effective nurse administrators must be knowledgeable about the costs of providing care to clients.

When 20 minutes are up, one member from each group should make a verbal report to the study group on how the assigned discipline influences nursing care.

The study group leader should summarize the discussion.

CASE STUDY

June Hill, R.N., works as a care provider on 3 East, a neurological unit at Western Hospital. June works in a case management system and coordinates care for a case load of clients, interacting with physicians, nurses, other health care workers, and outside agencies. She is viewed by her peers as a resource and is constantly sought for advice. June established the care management system on her unit, motivated her peers to "buy into" the new system, and convinced her manager that it was worthwhile. She enjoys her work and is continually influencing others to meet the goals she sets for client care.

Case Study Questions

1. Is June exhibiting leadership or management behaviors?
2. Can a nurse in a care provider position lead and/or manage?
3. What behaviors make a nurse an effective leader?
4. What behaviors make a nurse an effective manager?
5. Is June enacting the two basic roles of care provider and care manager?
6. From what disciplines might June have sought information during the development and implementation of the care management system?
7. What type of interdisciplinary collaboration would be important when constructing and implementing this new system?

Individual Activity: Understanding Interdisciplinary Contributions

Schedule time with a colleague from another discipline to have lunch to discuss a specific health care issue in your community. Clearly describe the issue you are interested in and then brainstorm different solutions or strategies to improve or resolve the issue. During the discussion write down the different ideas and strategies that were formulated.

Analyze the type of information provided by each participant and the strategies identified. Were more information and varied strategies formulated by a combination of disciplines to resolve the problem? What strengths did each disciplinary perspective provide to problem resolution? What approaches were taken to problem solving? What information and strategies were discipline-specific? Were ideas merged to create new solutions?

LEARNING RESOURCES

Discussion Questions

1. How can nurses use information from other disciplines to enhance their practice?
2. What is nursing administration, and what is the role of a practicing nurse in the provision and delivery of high-quality patient care?
3. How do leadership and management differ? Is it useful to possess both leadership and management behaviors?
4. Are all nurses in organizations involved in nursing administration? In what way?
5. What is the difference between a nurse executive, a nurse manager, and a nurse care provider?

Study Questions

True or False: Circle the correct answer.

T F 1. In acute care, the traditional medical model is predominant.

T F 2. The two basic roles of clinical nurses are to provide direct care and to supervise the care of clients.

T F 3. Conceptual acts include thinking, making decisions, and implementing plans.

T F 4. Nursing administration is the combination of leadership and management knowledge applied to nursing care delivery.

T F 5. Leadership and management are distinct ideas with no overlap.

T F 6. The two most common disciplines nurse managers synthesize are nursing and physiology.

T F 7. Nurse managers should not be concerned with organizational finances; they should focus on client care.

T F 8. The most effective nurses use a combination of leadership and management behaviors.

T F 9. Leadership is the coordination and integration of resources and plans to accomplish organizational objectives.

T F 10. Management is influencing people to accomplish goals and motivating followers by leading the way.

SUPPLEMENTAL READINGS

Christman, L.P. (1999). Creating nursing's future: Issues, opportunities, and challenges. *Nursing Administration Quarterly, 23(4)*, 99.

Flannery, T.P. (1999). Managing nursing assets: A primer on maximizing investment in people. *Nursing Administration Quarterly, 23(4)*, 35-42.

Henry, B., Arndt, C., Vincenti, M.D. & Marriner-Tomey, A. (1989). *Dimensions of Nursing Administration.* Blackwell Scientific Publication.

Morgan, J. (1999). Why does nursing practice need theory? *Assignment, 5(3)*, 29-31.

Rolfe, G. (1996). *Closing the theory-practice gap: A new paradigm for nursing*. Oxford: Butterworth-Heinemann Ltd.

Smith, M.C. (1993). The contribution of nursing theory to nursing administration practice. *Image: Journal of Nursing Scholarship 25(1)*, 63-67.

ANSWERS TO TEXT STUDY QUESTIONS

Chapter 1—Overview of Nursing Administration (p. 11)

1. **Does nursing administration differ from nursing practice? If so, how?**

   There is a distinct difference between nursing administration and nursing practice. Nursing practice uses specialized knowledge, science, and skill to provide client-based care. Nursing administration combines the knowledge of nursing practice with leadership and management theory to develop and organize care delivery systems, coordinate and manage client care, and to create a positive work environment.

2. **Are all nurses managers, or is management more properly confined to levels above staff nurses?**

   Although most nurses perform some tasks that would fall under the rubric of management, every nurse is not a nurse manager. As providers of care, nurses coordinate and direct care for a defined number of patients. The focus of a nurse manager is on the daily administration of nursing services provided by a group of nurses, 24 hours a day. According to Orem (1989), nurse managers are those who "manage nursing services for organizations."

3. **Are all nurses care coordinators? Is this the same as being a manager?**

   As the providers of care, nurses focus on the coordination of care provision to individuals or groups. This coordination may include activities such as direct care provision, providing access to health care services, initiating referrals, developing health promotion or risk reduction programs, and providing family support and education. The nurse manager concentrates on the coordination of health care employee activities to deliver quality care in a productive, cost-effective manner.

4. **Should a nurse follow a theory of administration as well as a theory of nursing?**

   As of yet, there is no one accepted theory of nursing administration. Nursing administration knowledge has been developed from theories of nursing, leadership, and management. Examples of theories that have been used in nursing administration include systems, bureaucratic, economic, management, organizational behavior, conflict, structural systems, and strategic choice. In addition, theories of motivation, chaos, conflict, organizational design, role, decision making, leadership, communication, and information processing have been applied in nursing administration.

The Health Care System

STUDY FOCUS

Countries create centralized or decentralized infrastructures for the delivery of health care services. The United States has a decentralized, complex, fragmented, costly health care system. Nursing is an integral part of the health care system and serves as the backbone or core function. General systems theory is useful in understanding health care services within organizations. Systems are sets of interacting elements that work together to accomplish specific goals. A key concept in systems theory is changes in one part of the system affect the other parts. Nursing services are a subset of the health care systems; and as such, there are interrelatedness and interdependence with other services. Chaos theory is useful in understanding transition that takes place within the health care system. Chaos theory provides new, nonlinear methods of thinking and learning. The flexibility and adaptability needed in chaos are needed for innovation, change, and creativity. Interactive planning is an approach useful in changing, chaotic environments. Interactive planning emphasizes participation among participants, a nonlinear view of relationships, and a focus on future outcomes.

The U.S. health care system is characterized by a lack of central planning, direction, and control. It is a blending of public and private stakeholders. The four basic functional components of the health care system are financing, insurance, delivery of care, and payment. There are four distinct phases in the U.S. health care system. First is the development of hospitals and the institutionalization of health care that occurred from 1850-1900. Second is the introduction of scientific methods that occurred from 1900-1940. Third is the growing interest in the social and organizational structure of health care that occurred from 1940 through the 1980s. Fourth is the limited resources, growth restrictions, and reorganization of the methods of financing and delivery of care in the early 1980s. The current emphasis in the U.S. health care system is on chronic illness and how genetics, personal lifestyles, and environmental hazards influence health.

Understanding the health care system is important for providing high-quality care at a reasonable cost to consumers. A health care system is composed of structures, organizations, and services designed to deliver professional health services to consumers. Integrated health care systems are merging to meet economic and community-based needs. These systems are interactive and interdependent health care units established through mergers, partnerships, and acquisitions. Integrated health care systems are formed in an attempt to increase efficiency and decrease cost by organizing a collection of health care providers to work interdependently and function as an open system, which adapts quickly to changes. All health care systems consist of five major components: production of resources, organizational structure, management, economic support, and delivery of services (Roemer, 1986). The five leading types of health care organizations are hospitals and other acute care institutions, ambulatory care, long-term care facilities, home health agencies, and mental health facilities (Kovner, 1990). With integrated health care systems, many of the health care organizations are partnering, merging, or acquiring facilities to compete effectively and provide community-based services.

Four key functions that help to explain health care delivery are financing, insurance, delivery method, and payment. Health care systems are being held accountable for the cost of services to provide quality care to clients. In the past, health care providers charged fixed fees for services provided. To contain costs, managed care systems were created. Managed care systems are health plans that offer a set group of health services for a set fee per client per year. In managed care, the term *per member* (or *enrollee*) *per month* refers to capitated payment. Managed care is not without problems: restricted choice in providers and services and financial incentives for physicians have created public fears. The emerging health care reform is targeting community-based health care systems to meet service needs at the local level. The building blocks of community health care management systems include population-based planning, integration of service systems, and continuous quality improvement.

In hospitals, prospective payment systems such as diagnosis-related groups are in place to limit and reduce costs for Medicare clients. The federal government funds two major programs: Medicare and Medicaid. Medicare is a two-part program of assistance with health care costs for individuals over 65 years of age and those who are disabled. Medicare Part A covers hospital costs and some nursing home care, and Part B covers physician services. Medicaid is a joint federal and state program administered by the states to pay for indigents' health care.

Despite efforts to contain costs, the total health care expenditures continue to rise at an alarming rate. The three categories of greatest total expenditure for health care are hospital care, physician fees, and prescription drugs. Prescription drugs have been growing at double-digit rates over the past few years as higher-priced drugs and consumer demand have fueled an increased prescription demand. Widespread concern exists that health care expenditures will continue to climb as the number of older citizens and cases of chronic illnesses increase. Changing ethnicity patterns, accelerating use of high technology, and escalating numbers of those infected with AIDS are also factors. Nurses will be challenged to provide community-based care to all clients, contain costs, and provide high-quality care. New roles are emerging for nurses with advanced practice degrees to perform primary care with emphasis on disease prevention, health promotion, and integration of health services across the continuum.

LEARNING TOOLS

Group Activity: Understanding Health care Systems

Purpose: To help you understand the U.S. health care system and to describe the impact of economics and governmental regulation on health care. The cost of health care in the U.S., the methods of controlling costs through integrated health care systems, and nursing's role in a changing health care environment will be examined.

Divide the study group into three smaller groups.

Assign each group to one of these topics: cost of health care in the U.S.; methods of controlling costs through integrated health care systems; or nursing's role in providing access to care for clients, containing costs, and ensuring high-quality care.

Each group should identify important points for the assigned topic (refer to the Huber textbook Chapter 2 for base information).

Provide 25 minutes for group discussion, and then have each group summarize its recommendations for large group discussion.

The study group leaders should serve as facilitators and summarize information.

CASE STUDY

Health care has become a big business in the United States and is very competitive in providing cost-effective care to clients. Stiff competition for market share and costs are weighed carefully before services are provided. Nurses are now in a position where they are expected not only to provide high-quality care at reasonable costs, but also to make recommendations that decrease costs while maintaining exemplary client care. Many factors influence the cost of health care for individuals. The three categories with the highest total expenditures include hospital costs, physician fees, and prescription drugs. Other factors that influence costs include the aging population, changing ethnicity patterns, and the increasing incidence of chronic illness. Government regulation, administrative costs for insurance handling, the lack of practice standardization and defensive medicine, and the overcapacity of hospital beds create further cost burdens in the United States. In addition, increasing consumer demands, the lack of healthy lifestyle practices, and new diseases and treatment contribute to rising costs.

Case Study Questions

1. How can nurses affect the cost of client care without compromising quality?
2. What strategies can nurses use to improve client care outcomes?
3. What cost factors do nurses control? What cost factors do nurses have influence over?
4. What could happen to the profession of nursing if nurses elect to ignore cost factors?

LEARNING RESOURCES

Discussion Questions

1. Can the five leading types of health care organizations (acute care, ambulatory care, long-term care, home health, and mental health facilities) form an integrated health care system? What are the advantages or disadvantages of integrated health care systems?

2. What is Medicare? What is Medicaid?
3. Health care expenditures continue to rise. What will happen to U.S. businesses if the cost of health insurance benefits continues to escalate?
4. Are nursing positions safe from downsizing and reductions in staff as health care agencies continue to cut costs? What strategies should nurses use to show their effect on patient outcomes?
5. How will nursing's role change as acute care agencies decrease in size and number and community-based care increases?
6. How can chaos theory provide a framework to analyze health care systems and develop strategic initiatives to effect change?

Study Questions

Matching: Write the letter of the correct response in front of each term.

_____ 1. Health care system
_____ 2. Integrated health care system
_____ 3. Medicare
_____ 4. Medicaid
_____ 5. Diagnosis-related group
_____ 6. Prospective payment system
_____ 7. Managed care

A. A payment system where prices are set before the service is provided
B. Federal government health care payment system for individuals over age 65
C. Federal and state health care payment program for indigent care
D. Structure and services to deliver health care to patients
E. Multiple agencies linked together to provide seamless health care
F. Categories of care based on severity of illness grouped according to medical conditions
G. Health plans that offer a set group of health services for a set fee per client per year

True or False: Circle the correct answer.

T F 1. Nurse administrators must balance access, cost, and quality to ensure excellent health care.
T F 2. Managed care indicates that one health care provider delivers all care to a caseload of clients.
T F 3. Frequently, hospital bills contain extra health care charges.
T F 4. Nursing care is the highest category in the gross national product of total health care expenditures in the United States.
T F 5. The cost of prescription drugs grew at double-digit rates over the past few years.

SUPPLEMENTAL READINGS

Bell, A. (1998). Public frustration with health care seen as biggest threat. *National Underwriter, 102(24)*, 3, 44.

Jacox, A. (1997). Determinants of who does what in health care. [Online]. Available at www.nursingworld.org/ojin/tpc5/tpc5_1.htm.

Kovner, A. (1990). *Health care delivery in the United States* (4th ed.). New York: Springer.

Roemer, M. (1986). *An introduction to the U.S. health care system* (2nd ed.). New York: Springer.

Sochalski, J. & Patrician, P. (1998). An overview of health care spending patterns in the United States: Using national data sources to explore trends in nursing service. [Online]. Available at www.nursingworld.org/ojin/tpc6/tpc6_1.htm.

Weber, D. (1997). Another dimension of patient-centered care delivery: Understanding the nature of demand. *The Health Care Manager, 15(4)*, 77-82.

Whitelaw, N.A. & Warden, G.L. (1999). Reexamining the delivery system as part of Medicare reform. *Health Affairs, 18(1)*, 132-143.

ANSWERS TO TEXT STUDY QUESTIONS

Chapter 2—The Health Care System (p. 30)

1. **What are the recent and projected developments in health care delivery? Are they changing?**

   The U.S. health care system has experienced major shifts in its attempt to provide care to clients with diverse health care needs. The health care system has shifted from institutional care where the emphasis was on acute illness and disease to a community-based approach with an emphasis on chronicity. In response to financial, political, and societal forces, the health care system is restructuring, redesigning, and integrating to reduce costs, manage resources, and maximize reimbursement. The continued development of reengineered systems, integrated networks, and new partnerships is projected to continue as the health care system and its professionals are required to become more accountable for quality outcomes and cost-effective services.

2. **What developments will challenge nurse leaders and managers the most?**

   Nurse leaders and managers will be challenged to create new roles that meet the dynamic nature of a new health care delivery system. As health care delivery shifts from the acute care environment into the community, nurses must be prepared for case management and advanced practice roles. In addition, expanded roles will require autonomous professionals to assess their leadership styles and to gain new skills and expertise in business, epidemiology, genetics, and informatics. Other challenges for nurse leaders include restructuring nursing education curricula to prepare nurses for practice in the new millennium, enhancing the marketability of professional nurses, and increasing the financial compensation for nurses.

3. **Where should nurses focus their vision and energy for the improvement of health services?**

   Nurses can improve health care services by focusing on the care of vulnerable populations such as the elderly, homeless, and the mentally ill, as well as increasing accessibility and availability of health care services to the underserved. Through the development of health promotion and risk reduction programs, nurses can address the multiplicity of needs in communities. Nurses are in a pivotal position to control health care costs through case management, advanced practice, program development, and client advocacy.

4. **Does the emphasis on cost containment overshadow nursing's role as a caring client advocate?**

   Cost containment is only one facet of a nurse's role. As a client advocate, nurses must bring attention to the millions of Americans who are uninsured, underinsured, and cannot afford the spiraling out-of-pocket expenses associated with our current health care system. Nurses are in a unique position to lead, manage, develop, and coordinate new care delivery systems that will bridge the gaps in health care, while containing costs.

5. **Should nursing control health care costs by slowing or halting nursing salary/benefit increases?**

   Inasmuch as nurses comprise the largest health care workforce, their salaries and benefits have been linked to health care expenditures and economic pressures. While the nursing profession has noted growth in starting salaries, in general salaries have remained compressed. Often, new graduates reach their maximum earning potential within seven years. In order to recruit individuals into the profession and enhance career longevity, nursing salaries must be analyzed and compared to the salaries of other professionals.

Professional Nursing Practice

STUDY FOCUS

The profession of nursing is defined by licensure laws and practice regulations in each state. The American Nurses Association provides leadership in defining nursing by publishing the definition of nursing, an ethical code, and standards of practice. The practice of nursing is broad and the scope and function of nursing practice is evolving. Nurses enact many different roles in practice. Examples include staff nurses, nurse practitioners, nurse anesthetists, nurse managers, midwives, case managers, and clinical nurse specialists.

Nurses perform many roles. *Role* is defined as the expected and associated behaviors of a specific job position (Hardy & Hardy, 1988). Nurses often perform the roles of clinician, educator, administrator, researcher, and consultant. One view of nurse's roles is twofold, that of a caregiver and integrator (McClure, 1991). The caregiver role is enacted in direct patient care, whereas the integrator role is a coordinating function to ensure a seamless integration of client care.

Is nursing a profession or an occupation? A *profession* is comprised of a system of roles that is socially defined. Professions hold contracts with society to provide services for the public good. In return for these essential services, society affords professionals (one who is engaged in a profession) higher prestige, income, and autonomy in their work. Professionalism is the extent to which an individual identifies with a profession and adheres to its standards. Members of society expect that professionals will uphold society's trust by possessing characteristics of expertise, engaging in rigorous academic preparation, and demonstrating commitment and responsible behavior. Professionalization is the process by which occupations set standards to move from nonprofessional to professional status.

The three most common criteria for a profession as identified by authors are service, knowledge, and autonomy. *Service* is providing society with essential activities; *knowledge* is the strong base of specialized education from which a profession practices; and professional *autonomy* is having authority over and accountability for one's decisions and activities. All professions have a code of ethics that guides practice. Professionalization of an occupation can be viewed on a continuum. An occupational group can move along the continuum from nonprofessional to semiprofessional to professional.

Nursing requires a high level of expertise, sophisticated decision-making, and a sense of service characteristic of professional groups. Problematic areas for nursing have been a lack of differentiated practice (multiple educational levels equated with one job assignment), the historical influence of religion and the military, nurses' own attitudes toward professionalization, and the fact that nursing is a profession in which most workers are women. Strong nursing leadership is required to assist in the professionalization of nursing. Nurses can use tools such as the Behavioral Inventory for Professionalism (Miller, Adams, & Beck, 1993) or a multidimensional instrument developed by Arthur (1995) to assess their level of professionalism. Nursing leaders must support autonomous nursing practice (job autonomy), continue to develop a strong nursing knowledge base, and use and contribute to nursing research, while being role models of professional behaviors. Using positive media images, educating the public about nursing's role in health care, acting altruistically in policymaking, and dressing and acting in a professional manner will also enhance the status and profession of nursing.

LEARNING TOOLS

Self-Assessment

Valiga Concept of Nursing Scale

Directions: The following statements I am attempting to ascertain the ideas which you currently hold about nursing as a profession, the role of the nurse, and the relationship of the nurse to the client and to the physician and other health team colleagues. Read each of the statements below carefully. Then for each statement please indicate whether you Strongly Agree (SA), Agree (A), are Undecided or Do Not Know (U), Disagree (D), or Strongly Disagree (SD) with the statement. Circle the one response that best expresses your opinion, and please be certain your response to each statement is clearly marked. There are no right or wrong answers, so please respond openly and honestly.

1. Nurses must be willing to enter with clients those health-related situations which patients cannot face alone. SA A U D SD

2. Nursing is concerned with helping people maximize their health potential in their particular life situation. SA A U D SD

3. Overt action, directed by logical thought, toward meeting the client's need for help constitutes the practice of clinical nursing. SA A U D SD

4. Nurses must assume responsibility for diagnosing and treating human responses to actual or potential illnesses. SA A U D SD

5. The independent functions of nurses include supervising the care of clients, observing and recording, supervising nonprofessional personnel, and health teaching. SA A U D SD

6. Nursing must be concerned equally with the prevention of disease and the conservation of health. SA A U D SD

7. Nursing is an expression of one's commitment to others. SA A U D SD

8. Nurses must be involved actively in professional organizations. SA A U D SD

9. There is definitely a right and a wrong way to do things and approach nursing situations. SA A U D SD

10. Nurses should make written or verbal contacts with all appropriate persons to assure continuity of nursing care for clients. SA A U D SD

11. The uniqueness of nursing lies in the reasons for what nurses do in society, rather than in the specific tasks they perform. SA A U D SD

12. Nurses should be concerned primarily with giving physical care to clients as directed by the physician. SA A U D SD

13. There should be only one nursing theory. SA A U D SD

14. Evaluation of the work of their peers and other nursing personnel should be a responsibility of nurses. SA A U D SD

15. Nurses must follow doctor's orders without question. SA A U D SD

16. Nurses should be free to practice nursing as they define it within the scope of professional autonomy. SA A U D SD

17. Nurses should assume responsibility for the total nursing care of a caseload of clients. SA A U D SD

18. Nurses should update their knowledge through lifelong continuing education. SA A U D SD

19. Nurses must control and direct their own practice. SA A U D SD

20. Nurses should be responsible for conducting nursing care conferences routinely. SA A U D SD

21. Nurses must be aware that people who require their assistance are helpless and dependent and usually need to be told what to do. SA A U D SD

22. Nurses have a responsibility for discussing the proposed medical plan of care with the physician so it can be adjusted, if possible, to be more acceptable to the client. SA A U D SD

23. Nurses must assume responsibility for reviewing and evaluating care provided by nursing peers. SA A U D SD

24. Nurses must take deliberate action to attain independence in nursing situations. SA A U D SD

25. Nurses must not hesitate to assume the role of leader of the health care team when the client's problems are best met by nurses. SA A U D SD

Scoring: Each individual receives a score of +2 for each item with which they strongly agree, +1 for each item with which they agree, 0 for each item about which they were unsure, –1 for each item with which they disagreed, and –2 for each item with which they strongly disagreed. The minimum score is –50 and the maximum score is +50. The higher the + score, the stronger the professional view.

(Courtesy of Theresa M. Valiga, RN, EdD, Dean and Professor, School of Nursing, Fairfield University, Fairfield, Connecticut.)

CASE STUDY

Kay is a staff nurse on the oncology unit at Zimmer Hospital in Austin, Texas. She has been a registered nurse for three years. Kay graduated with a baccalaureate degree in nursing and has continued to enroll in one course per term toward her master's degree. Kay is active in the Texas Nurses Association, and she is the secretary for the local Oncology Nurses Association. She subscribes to two nursing journals and attends continuing educational programs at the hospital. She enjoys her work and volunteers for clinical projects.

Case Study Questions

1. Does Kay demonstrate behaviors that indicate she is career- or occupation-oriented?
2. What characteristics of a professional nurse does Kay demonstrate?
3. What types of master's degree programs in nursing may Kay elect to pursue?

LEARNING RESOURCES

Discussion Questions

1. What is nursing's scope of practice? What are some examples of nursing roles that illustrate that "nursing" has a broad and evolving scope of practice?
2. What are the twofold roles of nursing that McClure identifies? Give examples of each role.
3. What are the categories on the continuum of professionalization? Which category does nursing fit?

4. Does nursing fit the major three categories of a profession (service, knowledge, and autonomy)?
5. How does advanced nursing practice fit into professional nursing practice?
6. What barriers are there in nursing's process of professionalization? What driving forces influence nursing's process of professionalization?
7. How have nursing's historical influences (religion and the military) and gender issues influenced nursing's quest toward professionalization?

Study Questions

Matching: Write the letter of the correct response in front of each term.

_____ 1. Professionalism
_____ 2. Profession
_____ 3. Professional
_____ 4. Professionalization
_____ 5. Differentiated practice
_____ 6. Altruism
_____ 7. Job autonomy
_____ 8. Professional autonomy

A. Comprised of a system of roles that are socially defined
B. One educational level for one job assignment
C. The authority and accountability for one's work
D. Individual and collective authority and accountability
E. Selfless concern and service to others
F. One who is engaged in a profession
G. The extent to which an individual identifies and adheres to professional standards
H. Process where occupations change in the direction of a profession

True or False: Circle the correct answer.

T F 1. McClure defines nursing's roles as caregiver and integrator.

T F 2. The scope of nursing is changing and evolving.

REFERENCES

Arthur, D. (1995). Measurement of the professional self-concept of nurses: Developing a measurement instrument. *Nursing Education Today, 15(5)*, 328-335.

Hardy, M.E. & Hardy, W.L. (1988). Role stress and role strain. In M.E. Hardy & M.E. Conway (Eds.), *Role Theory: Perspectives for Health Professionals*, (2nd Ed.), pp. 159-239. Norwalk, CT: Appleton & Lange.

McClure, M.L. (1991). Introduction. In I.E. Goertzen (Ed.), *Differentiating Nursing Practice in the Twenty-First Century*, pp. 1-9. Kansas City, MO: American Academy of Nursing.

Miller, B., Adams, D. & Beck, L. (1993). A behavioral inventory for professionalism in nursing. *Journal of Professional Nursing, 9(5)*, 290-295.

SUPPLEMENTAL READINGS

Barger, S.E. (1999). Professional practice: Partnerships for practice—a necessity in the new millennium. *Journal of Professional Nursing, 15(4)*, 20.

Chitty, K.K. (1993). Defining profession. In Chitty, K. (Ed.), Professional nursing concepts and challenge (pp. 113-123). Philadelphia: W.B. Saunders.

Chitty, K.K. (1993). Professional socialization. In Chitty, K. (Ed.), *Professional Nursing Concepts and Challenge*, pp. 136-155. Philadelphia: W.B. Saunders.

Fosbinder, D., Parsons, R.J., Dwore, R.B., Murray, B., Gustafson, G., Dalley, K. & Vorderer, L.H. (1999). Effectiveness of nurse executives: Measurement of role factors and attitudes. *Nursing Administration Quarterly, 23(3)*, 52-62.

Lindeke, L.L. & Block, D.E. (1998). Maintaining professional integrity in the midst of interdisciplinary collaboration. *Nursing Outlook, 46(5)*, 213-218.

Purrell, L.D. (1999). Heath care managers' and administrators' roles, functions, and responsibilities. *Nursing Administration Quarterly, 23(3)*, 26-37.

ANSWERS TO TEXT STUDY QUESTIONS

Chapter 3—Professional Nursing Practice (p. 46)

1. **On what basis can nursing argue that it is a profession?**

   The three most commonly cited criteria of a profession include service, knowledge, and autonomy. Nursing can argue that it is a profession on the basis of client service, commitment, and responsibility. It has a long history of socially sanctioned service that dates back to the days of Florence Nightingale and the Crimean War. Meeting the criteria of knowledge and autonomy has been more problematic. Nurses are beginning to engage in autonomous practice through expanded roles and advanced practice. As a knowledge-based discipline, nursing incorporates systematic theory and specialized skills to advance the welfare of society. Continued efforts to develop the scientific body of knowledge that guides professional nursing practice will help to solidify its status as a profession.

2. **How close to a true profession is nursing today? Which elements are progressing the fastest?**

   Contemporary nursing is close to achieving true professional status. Nursing has fulfilled its obligation to service and is making progress in the areas of developing specialized knowledge and in establishing control over practice. The actualization of the advanced practice nurse role, the establishment of professional conduct standards, and the development of nursing-sensitive outcomes are examples of important accomplishments that will facilitate the recognition of nursing as a legitimate profession.

3. **Should nurses put their energy into activities of professionalism?**

   It is important that nurses have an organized voice to represent their values, concerns, and contributions. Active involvement in professions can formulate and frame professional identity, provide opportunities for self-actualization, and enhance self-esteem. Participation in professional organizations and associations may serve to stabilize the workforce and serve as a strategy to recruit individuals into the nursing profession.

4. **What strategy or strategies can nursing use to move nursing's professionalization to full professional status?**

   If nursing is to actualize a status as a true profession it must adapt and adhere to minimal standards of education and practice. A baccalaureate degree in nursing must serve as the basic preparation for professional nursing practice and a master's degree in nursing as the prerequisite for advance practice and leadership positions. Professional nurses need to be distinguished from nonprofessional nurses by job classification, responsibility, and financial remuneration. Additionally, if nursing is to achieve full professional status it must have the solidarity of its members and their commitment to a single, strong organization that will represent professional nursing.

5. **Should nurses care about image and appearance? If so, why?**

   If nurses are to convince themselves, professional colleagues, and the public that they are professionals, it is imperative that nurses present themselves in a professional manner. The image that nurses project influences the response, regard, and respect that they are afforded.

6. **What is the most prevalent media stereotype of nurses today? How could this be changed?**

   The media continues to depict nurses in a disparaging and degrading manner. Nurses are often stereotyped as amoral, uncaring women. This negative image of nursing may be changed through organized protests, media campaigns that accurately describe nurses' unique contribution to health care, and the dissemination of nursing research into the community. These initiatives may serve to change the image of nurses from one that is maligned to one that is respected and admired.

7. **Do nurses need to act and look professional to give a professional impression?**

   Nurses must act and behave in a professional manner if they are to be perceived as serious and legitimate health care professionals by colleagues, clients, and reimbursement agencies.

   Professional impressions are formulated based on conduct, action, and demeanor.

8. **Can you design the "ideal" nursing uniform—one that nurses like and find comfortable and practical and yet clients can identify?**

   The "ideal" nursing uniform is one that allows the nurse to function in a professional manner. Depending on the given situation, it may be a scrub outfit, a white uniform, or a business suit. The ideal nursing uniform does not depend on a given color, fabric, or style; for it is the nurse that makes the uniform, not the uniform that makes the nurse.

Leadership Principles

STUDY FOCUS

Leadership is crucial in health care where relentless change is affecting the organization, delivery, and financing of services. *Leadership* is the process of influencing people to accomplish goals by inspiring confidence and support among followers. Skill at interpersonal relationships and applying the problem-solving process are fundamental to leadership. Strong leadership empowers individuals and instills them with a belief and confidence in their ability to achieve and succeed. In contrast, *management* is the process of influencing employees to work toward the organization's goals by integrating resources through planning, organizing, coordinating, directing, and controlling. Managers obtain power to accomplish objectives from their position and title (Trott & Windsor, 1999).

The new role of leader/manager is to facilitate the development of effective support systems to generate efficiencies directed to improving processes. *Leadership styles* are combinations of task and relationship behaviors used to influence others to accomplish goals. *Followership* is an interpersonal process of participating by following. *Empowerment* is the giving of authority, responsibility, and freedom to act. Empowerment instills a belief and confidence in one's ability to achieve. There are three levels of leadership. The individual level of leadership involves activities such as mentoring, coaching, and motivating others. The group level of leadership involves building teams and resolving conflict. The organizational level of leadership involves building culture.

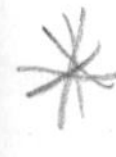

The five interwoven aspects of leadership are the leader, the follower, the situation, the communication process, and the goals (Kison, 1989). Leaders' values, experiences, skills, and expertise are important ingredients in their ability to lead effectively. Transactional leaders function in a caretaker role focusing on day-to-day operations. Transformational leaders motivate followers to perform to their full potential and provide a sense of direction. Followers either reject or accept the leader and determine their own level of participation and the leader's power within the group. Followers may exhibit the Pygmalion effect; that is, acting according to what the leader expects. The situation includes the work to be done, control systems, available resources, the amount of time, the level of interaction, and the external forces affecting the type of decision task. The communication process is the vital means for leaders and followers to send and receive clear messages, both verbal and nonverbal, through formal and informal channels. The goals include the organizational, personal, and professional goals of the leader and follower.

Leadership characteristics include taking risks, communicating a vision, empowering the followership, mastering change, and motivating groups to achieve goals. Effective leaders know that a leader is someone who has followers, leaders are visible and set examples, and leadership is not rank, but responsibility. Leadership is not popularity; leadership is results. There are many leadership theories, including attitudinal leadership, situational leadership, Fiedler's contingency, and Hersey and Blanchard's Tridimensional Leader Effectiveness Model. Three styles of leadership are authoritarian, democratic, and laissez-faire. Authoritarian leadership refers to directive and controlling behaviors by which the leader in isolation determines policies and makes decisions, and then orders subordinates to carry out the tasks or work. This style is helpful in crisis situations. Democratic leadership is a team approach whereby the leader facilitates and coordinates material and human resources and shares responsibility for decision mak-

ing and quality improvement. All members of the group are encouraged to actively participate in a cohesive fashion to accomplish team objectives. The democratic leadership style is useful when professional staff work together to establish and meet goals. A laissez-faire leader is one who does not interfere in decision making or policy setting through preference or incompetence. This style may be useful with highly qualified professionals who work well in teams to accomplish established goals.

Nurse leaders are challenged in today's rapidly changing practice environment. They need to exert effective leadership in order to affect positive organizational and individual productivity. At a national level, nurses, representing the largest health care profession in the United States, need to band together to provide leadership and direction in health care delivery. Nurses must also provide leadership in advocating positive health care practices for clients and communities. The nursing leadership challenge is to develop strategies that help followers cope with change and develop the ability to adapt in a positive and productive way.

LEARNING TOOLS

Task Orientation and People Orientation Leadership Questionnaire: An Assessment of Style

Purpose: To assess your leadership style in the areas of task and people orientation and to assess your leadership style profile in relation to autocratic, shared (democratic), and laissez-faire leadership.

Directions: The following items describe aspects of leadership behavior. Respond to each item according to the way you would most likely act if you were the leader of a work group. Circle whether you would most likely behave in the described way: always (A), frequently (F), occasionally (O), seldom (S), or never (N).

A F O S N 1. I would most likely act as the spokesman of the group.

A F O S N 2. I would encourage overtime work.

A F O S N 3. I would allow members complete freedom in their work.

A F O S N 4. I would encourage the use of uniform procedures.

A F O S N 5. I would permit the members to use their own judgment in solving problems.

A F O S N 6. I would stress being ahead of competing groups.

A F O S N 7. I would speak as a representative of the group.

A F O S N 8. I would needle members for greater effort.

A F O S N 9. I would try out my ideas in the group.

A F O S N 10. I would let the members do their work the way they think best.

A F O S N 11. I would be working hard for a promotion.

A F O S N 12. I would tolerate postponement and uncertainty.

A F O S N 13. I would speak for the group if there were visitors present.

A F O S N 14. I would keep the work moving at a rapid pace.

A F O S N 15. I would turn the members loose on a job and let them go to it.

A F O S N 16. I would settle conflicts when they occur in the group.

A F O S N 17. I would get swamped by details.

A F O S N 18. I would represent the group at outside meetings.

A F O S N 19. I would be reluctant to allow the members any freedom of action.

A F O S N 20. I would decide what should be done and how it should be done.

A F O S N 21. I would push for increased production.

A F O S N 22. I would let some members have authority which I could keep.

A F O S N 23. Things would usually turn out as I had predicted.

A F O S N 24. I would allow the group a high degree of initiative.

A F O S N 25. I would assign group members to particular tasks.

A F O S N 26. I would be willing to make changes.

A F O S N 27. I would ask the members to work harder.

A F O S N 28. I would trust the group members to exercise good judgment.

A F O S N 29. I would schedule the work to be done.

A F O S N 30. I would refuse to explain my actions.

A F O S N 31. I would persuade others that my ideas are to their advantage.

A F O S N 32. I would permit the group to set its own pace.

A F O S N 33. I would urge the group to beat its previous record.

A F O S N 34. I would act without consulting the group.

A F O S N 35. I would ask that group members follow standard rules and regulations.

T______ P______

Scoring: *First:* Circle the item number for items 8, 12, 17, 18, 19, 30, 34, and 35. Write the number 1 in front of a circled item number if you responded S (seldom) or N (never) to that item. *Second:* Write a number 1 in front of item numbers not circled if you responded A (always) or F (frequently). Circle the number 1s which you have written in front of the following items: 3, 5, 8, 10, 15, 18, 19, 22, 24, 26, 28, 30, 32, 34, and 35. *Third:* Count the circled number 1s. This is your score for concern for people. Record the score in the blank following the letter P at the end of the questionnaire. *Fourth:* Count the uncircled number 1s. This is your score for concern for task. Record this number in the blank following the letter T.

Awareness of your leadership style will help you to tailor your responses in personal or work situations. You will be able to compare your perception of how people- and task-oriented you are with a score of how you respond in specific situations. The next step is to determine if your score matches your desired response and determine whether to continue your present leadership style or to make changes to become more participate (if you score high on autocratic leadership style) or more directive (if you score high on laissez-faire leadership style).

Task-Orientation and People-Orientation Leadership Style Profile Sheet

Directions: To determine your style of leadership, mark your score on the concern for task dimension (T) on the left-hand arrow below. Next, move to the right-hand arrow and mark your score on the concern for people dimension (P). Draw a straight line that intersects the P and T scores. The point at which the line crosses the shared leadership arrow indicates your score on that dimension.

Shared Leadership Results from Balancing Concern for Task and Concern for People

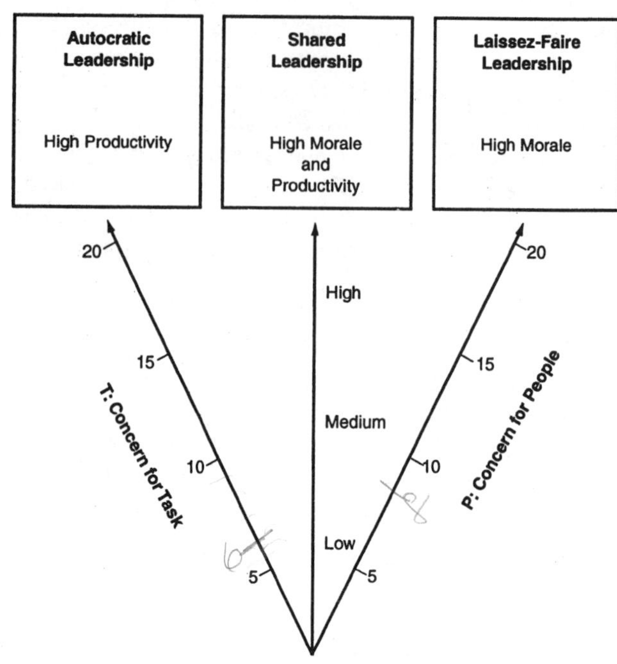

 The T-P Leadership Questionnaire was adapted from Sergiovanni, Metzcus, and Burden's revision of the Leadership Behavior Description Questionnaire, *American Educational Research Journal* 6 (1969), pages 62-79.

CASE STUDY

Jennifer is the nurse manager of a 68-bed respiratory unit with 95 employees. Jennifer tailors her leadership style according to the employees' needs, experience, and situation. She is helping a graduate nurse who is in orientation to learn how to use the documentation forms. Jennifer provides detailed instructions to the new nurse, explaining step-by-step the process for documentation. In another situation, Jennifer asks a seasoned clinical nurse to take responsibility for the total quality improvement process. She provides the nurse with information and offers to assist any time the clinical nurse needs consultation. Jennifer promotes Susan, a clinical nurse, to a 3-11 charge position. Since this is Susan's first management experience, Jennifer is providing a structured orientation, but is giving Susan the opportunity to seek out the information she needs and to design learning objectives to meet her needs.

Case Study Questions

1. What type of leadership theory is Jennifer using?
2. What are the benefits of changing the leadership style based on the employee's experience, knowledge, and situation?
3. What is the relationship between followership and leadership?
4. What levels of leadership is Jennifer engaging in the work environment? Provide examples for each level.

LEARNING RESOURCES

Discussion Questions

1. Is a clinical nurse a leader?
2. What are the characteristics of effective leaders? Identify an effective leader.
3. What is situational leadership? Are the three styles of leadership—authoritarian, democratic, and laissez-faire—interchangeable? What are the differences?
4. How can nursing as a profession exhibit leadership in defining policy for health care delivery?
5. According to Kouzes & Posner, what are the five practices common to exceptional leadership achievements?

Study Questions

Fill-in-the-Blank: Identify the appropriate leadership style for the following situations.

1. A code has been called. Which leadership style is most effective in this situation? ________________

   ____
2. The nursing record is being revised. Which leadership style is most appropriate? ________________

   ____
3. Nurses, physicians, dietitians, and social workers are working together to increase patient services in a hospital. Which leadership style is useful? ____________

   ____

True or False: Circle the correct answer.

T F 1. Two critical skills in leadership are interpersonal and problem-solving skills.

T F 2. Followership is a process whereby leaders participate in group decisions.

T F 3. Empowerment is the ability to lead a group successfully.

T F 4. Important skills for leading include diagnosing, adapting, and communicating.

T F 5. Situational leaders tailor their leadership style based on the employee, experience, and situation.

T F 6. Laissez-faire leadership entails minimal participation and directing by the leader resulting in high productivity.

T F 7. A transactional leader is one who motivates employees to their full potential.

T F 8. The new role of leader/manager is to facilitate the development of effective support systems to generate efficiencies directed to improving processes.

T F 9. Popularity is leadership.

T F 10. Leadership is not rank, but responsibility.

REFERENCES

Kison, C. (1989). Leadership: How, who and what? Nursing Management, 20(11), 72-74.

Trott, M.C. & Windsor, K. (1999). Leadership effectiveness: How do you measure up? *Nursing Economics*, *7(4)*, 204-207, 230.

SUPPLEMENTAL READINGS

Curtin, L.L. (1997). How—and how not—to be a transformational leader. *Nursing Management*, *23(2)*, 7-8.

Hotko, B. & Van Dyke, D. (1998). Peer review: Strengthening leadership skills. *Nursing Management*, *29(4)*, 41-44.

Kouzes, J. & Posner, B. (1988). The leadership practices inventory. San Diego, CA: Pfeiffer & Company.

Laschinger, H.K., Wong, C., McMahon, L. & Kaufmann, C. (1999). Leader behavior impact on staff nurse empowerment, job tension, and work effectiveness. *Journal of Nursing Administration*, *29(5)*, 28-39.

Stahl, D. (1998). Subacute care: Creating alternatives. Manage, lead, inspire. *Nursing Management*, *29(10)*, 18-21.

ANSWERS TO TEXT STUDY QUESTIONS

Chapter 4—Leadership Principles (p. 72)

1. **How would you describe a leader? Identify one person who personifies leadership.**

   Leadership entails influencing others to accomplish goals. It is an interactional process that involves motivation, communication, and innovation to influence and engage individuals in goal attainment. In other words, people are the focus of leaders, whereas organizational goals and objectives are the primary focus of managers. Managers are concerned with systems and structures, as well as the management of organizational resources. Florence Nightingale was a leader in nursing. Her visionary leadership, combined with her willingness to take risks and to actively engage the environment, helped to shape the profession of nursing. Who do you know that personifies leadership?

2. **What are the important qualities of leadership?**

   Effective leaders are dynamic, visionary individuals. They are productive, responsible, and visible to their followers. Leaders demonstrate strong interpersonal skills to influence, motivate, and guide groups of individuals toward goal achievement. The ability to be a change agent, take calculated risks, build team relationships, to lead by example, and to develop new cultures are important qualities of a leader. When these qualities are evident in leaders, followers perceive them as courageous, honest, and trustworthy.

3. **What is the best way to learn leadership skills?**

   The best way to learn leadership skills is through education and practice. Nurses can become more effective leaders by analyzing their interactions with others, diagnosing areas for improvement, and practicing the skills needed to enhance their leadership ability. Diagnosing a problematic situation, adapting one's behavior to match the situation, and communicating clearly can improve leadership effectiveness.

4. **Who are the leaders in nursing?**

   Two types of leaders in nursing include transactional and transformational leaders. Transactional nursing leaders work with the existing organizational culture. They maintain the status quo by coordinating and managing the environment, and by focusing on the day-to-day operations. In contrast, transformational leaders influence and change the organization's culture. They use innovation, charisma, individual consideration, and intellectual stimulation to effect change.

5. **Can you be a leader in nursing?**

   Many leaders are needed in the profession of nursing. Nurses can learn and practice leadership skills that will enable them to be effective leaders. According to Kouzes and Posner (1990), exceptional leadership practices include challenging the process, inspiring a vision, enabling others, modeling the way, and encouraging the heart.

6. **What are some examples of leadership opportunities or challenges that you have faced? How did you handle them?**

   Leaders must assess the group they are working with, match leadership behaviors to the environment, and adapt their style to accommodate the group's needs. Groups take on a personality, and a skilled leader will be able to ascertain the maturity and the readiness level of the group. The selected leadership style will be different depending on the composition of the group. A more knowledgeable, experienced, and mature group will present different opportunities and challenges than a less experience group. What opportunities and challenges have you encountered as both a leader and as a group member?

7. **What is a good follower?**

   Followers are essential because they either accept or reject the leader, and determine the scope of the leader's power. While there are varying degrees of followership engagement, effective followers demonstrate initiative and independent thinking. In addition, effective followers are responsible, competent, and committed individuals that should be nurtured, developed, and valued as assets to the organization.

8. **What is your favorite leadership style? Followership style?**

   Leadership styles are a combination of task and relationship behaviors used to influence others to accomplish goals. A leader may select behaviors among three distinct leadership styles: authoritarian, democratic, and laissez-faire. If you primarily demonstrate directive behaviors, then authoritarian is your leadership style. Behaviors reflecting a relationship and person orientation indicate a democratic style, whereas behaviors that promote independence and freedom reflect a laissez-faire leadership style. It's important to recognize that one leadership style is not better than any other; each has its own advantages and disadvantages, depending on the situation. Followership styles include the "sheep" who lack initiative, a sense of responsibility, and critical thinking; "yes-people" who lack enterprise and yield to the opinions of others; and "alienated" followers who are independent and critical thinkers, but passively resist open opposition.

Management Principles

STUDY FOCUS

Management is the coordination and integration of resources through planning, organizing, directing, and controlling to accomplish specific organizational goals and objectives. *Nursing management* is coordinating and integrating nursing resources by applying the management process to organize and deliver high-quality client care to individuals, groups, and communities. The *management process* is composed of four steps: planning, organizing, directing, and controlling. A major task of management is to link the staff at the bottom of the organization with those at the top. Nurse managers must continuously balance two important—and at times competing—needs: those of the staff for growth and those of the organization for viability.

Planning for the needs of individuals and the organization is complex and requires time and skill. *Strategic planning* is a long-term process that provides direction and purpose for the organization. *Tactical planning* is typically a short-term process that focuses on the specific details of activities necessary to accomplish the broad organizational goals. In order to accomplish goals, the manager must organize the integration and coordination of resources. *Organization* is the mobilization of the human, financial, and material resources of the agency to achieve established goals. *Directing* employees by motivating and providing leadership is essential to goal accomplishment. Nurse managers must know the scope of nursing practice to assign and delegate tasks to appropriate personnel. After the nurse manager has assigned work to staff and goals have been accomplished, evaluation of the outcomes is necessary. *Controlling* refers to examining the results of activities (outcomes) in light of a predetermined standard for the purpose of quality control and then taking corrective actions when necessary.

A *nurse manager* is a registered nurse who holds 24-hour accountability for management of the health care unit(s). The nurse manager's role is complex and varied, encompassing multiple diverse tasks, many of which require immediate action. The components of the nurse manager role include managing care delivery, managing resources, developing personnel, complying with regulatory and professional standards, and fostering interdisciplinary and collaborative relationships. Mintzberg (1975) identifies ten important role behaviors for managers which he categorizes into three role sets. The role sets are interpersonal (figurehead, leader, and liaison), informational (monitor, disseminator, and spokesperson), and decisional (entrepreneur, disturbance handler, resource allocator, and negotiator).

Managing difficult individuals is a challenging task for any manager. Difficult individuals may exhibit negative attitudes or behaviors. Lewis-Ford (1993) describes the following categories of difficult people: Sherman tanks, snipers, exploders, bulldozers, balloons, clams, negative nabobs, complainers, and stallers. Tactics to use with these individuals include trying to understand their behavior, preparing yourself psychologically to interact with them, and selecting disciplinary measures, if necessary.

Nurse managers who are skilled in coordination and integration are valuable resources in the changing health care environment. They are able to adopt new flexible strategies and structures to enhance productivity and quality patient care while meeting community health care needs. Nurse managers who successfully manage large numbers of employees and balance complex job demands are developing creative strategies to proactively manage an increasingly complex, turbulent health care environment. Nurse managers are adapting systems, developing strategic plans, and fostering interdisciplinary collaboration, and partnering with community members while integrating and reconfiguring health care services.

LEARNING TOOLS

Self-Assessment

Purpose: To explore your strengths and areas for improvement in leadership and management behaviors.

Directions: Circle the option that reflects how often you engage in the leadership or management behavior listed.

Management Self Assessment Study Guide

A=Always M=Most of the time S=Some of the time O=Occasionally N=Never

1. Enjoys being visible and interacting at work.
   A M S O N
2. Communicates vision to others effectively.
   A M S O N
3. Is able to motivate others to accomplish goals.
   A M S O N
4. Seeks out new resources to resolve problems.
   A M S O N
5. Consistently evaluates outcomes.
   A M S O N
6. Coordinates client care.
   A M S O N
7. Plans daily activities and accomplishes them.
   A M S O N
8. Makes assignments.
   A M S O N
9. Sets goals for self.
   A M S O N
10. Negotiates with others to accomplish tasks.
    A M S O N
11. Is comfortable with change.
    A M S O N
12. Initiates change.
    A M S O N
13. Communicates effectively with others.
    A M S O N
14. Develops strong peer relationships.
    A M S O N
15. Is able to resolve conflicts.
    A M S O N
16. Establishes information networks.
    A M S O N
17. Feels comfortable making decisions in conditions of extreme ambiguity.
    A M S O N
18. Guards own perspective and avoids taking the behavior personally.
    A M S O N
18. Enjoys building teams and working cooperatively.
    A M S O N
19. Consistently meets deadlines.
    A M S O N
20. Is able to manage multiple priorities.
    A M S O N

Scoring: Identify the items that you marked Always or Most of the Time. These are the leadership and management behaviors in which you are strong and excel. Now, identify the items that you marked Some of the Time, Occasionally, or Never. These are the leadership and management behaviors that are areas for improvement or growth. By working on these areas you can improve your leadership skills.

CASE STUDY

Ruth Anne is a nurse manager of an oncology unit for Middle View Hospital in North Dakota. Ruth Anne has been a manager for 15 years and enjoys the role. She is proud of the fact that she has never once been over budget at year end, has maintained a high productivity level, and has a stable core staff. Ruth Anne is very detail-oriented and organized. Ruth Anne conscientiously follows policies and procedures, and implements new programs according to protocol. She meets monthly with the director of the medical/surgical areas and keeps her abreast of any changes in the unit. Ruth Anne is open to innovations that the director asks her to initiate. Ruth Anne treats all employees equitably and follows the personnel handbook for any human resource issue.

Case Study Questions

1. Does Ruth Anne exhibit managerial or leadership behaviors?
2. What management behaviors does she exhibit?
3. With the changing health care environment, what types of leadership and management behaviors will be important for Ruth Anne to use to improve performance and efficiencies on the oncology unit?

LEARNING RESOURCES

Discussion Questions

1. What are the legal aspects of management in the nurse manager's role?

2. What are some categories of difficult people? What are some effective methods to manage difficult people?
3. What is the management process? What is involved in each of the four steps?
4. What is the role of a nurse manager? What is the nature of managerial work?
5. How do management and leadership differ? Are there similarities between leadership and management?

Study Questions

True or False: Circle the correct answer.

T F 1. Leadership is more important than management in a turbulent health care environment.

T F 2. Transformational leaders focus on the maintenance of quality and quantity of performance.

T F 3. Transformational leadership is necessary in periods of growth, change, and crisis.

T F 4. Management is focused on tasks and accomplishing organizational goals.

T F 5. Nursing management is the coordination and integration of resources using a political and computer science process.

T F 6. The traditional management functions include planning, organizing, controlling, and coordinating.

T F 7. Tactical planning is a broad-range process of establishing the purpose and direction of the organization.

T F 8. Management is a discipline that uses a set of tools to achieve desired outcomes.

T F 9. Organizing is determining the long- and short-term objectives and the corresponding actions taken to achieve objectives.

T F 10. Nurse managers usually have 24-hour accountability for the coordination and delivery of care.

REFERENCES

Lewis-Ford, B. (1993). Management techniques: Coping with difficult people. *Nursing Management, 24(3)*, 36-38.

Mintzberg, H. (1975). The manager's job: Folklore and fact. In M. Matteson and J. Ivancevich (Eds.), *Management Classics* (3rd ed.) (pp. 63-85). Plano, TX: Business Publications.

SUPPLEMENTAL READINGS

McBain, R. (1999). Human resources management: Resistance, fairness and satisfaction. *Manager Update, 11(1)*, 22-30.

Schmidt, D.Y. (1999). Financial and operational skills for nurse managers. *Nursing Administration Quarterly, 23(4)*, 16-28.

Shearer, R., Davidhizar, R. & Dowd, S.B. (1998). Humor: No material manager should be without it. *Hospital Material Management Quarterly, 20(1)*, 29-36.

Valadez, A.M. & Sportsman, S. (1999). Environmental management: Principles from quantum theory. *Journal of Professional Nursing, 15(4)*, 209-213.

ANSWERS TO TEXT STUDY QUESTIONS

Chapter 5—Management Principles (p. 93)

1. **Which is more important: leadership or management?**

   It is important to recognize that leadership and management are equally vital processes. The focus of each process is different, though their outcomes may be interrelated. How important one process is over the other depends on what is needed at the time and the context in which it occurs.

2. **Why is management important to a nurse?**

   As managers of care, management is an important concept to nurses. Nurses coordinate and deliver health services to clients. Nursing management is the coordination and integration of nursing resources to accomplish care provision through application of the management process.

3. **Are middle managers going to become obsolete?**

   According to the American Organization of Nurse Executives (AONE) (1992), nurse managers are individuals who have 24-hour accountability for the management of client care unit(s) or area(s) within a health care institution. Essential components of the nurse manager's role are the management of human, fiscal, and other resources needed for nursing practice and care delivery. The complexity of the nurse management role and the skills necessary to manage multiskilled, cross-functional work groups will continue to intensify as organizations reconfigure, restructure, and integrate.

4. **How do Mintzberg's ten roles differ for nurses at different positions in the hierarchical bureaucracy?**

   Mintzberg (1975) identified ten roles that describe a manager's role. The three interpersonal roles—figurehead, leader, and liaison—evolve from the formal authority and status of the management position. Informational roles include monitor, disseminator, and spokesperson, and the decision-making roles include entrepreneur, disturbance handler, resource allocator, and negotiator. Engagement in these three roles, including the amount of time involved and the type of individuals with which they interact, depends on whether one is a care manager, nurse manager, or nurse executive in the hierarchical bureaucracy. Care managers provide direct care to clients and make clinical decisions through interactions with clients, physicians, and colleagues. The nurse manager focuses on the coordination of care delivery and manages interactions with employees and administrators, as well as clients and families. The focus of the nurse executive is on strategic management, policy formation, and service delivery analysis and trending. Nurse executives interact most frequently with other administrators, managers, and board members.

5. **Is it easier for nurses to change to a new managerial role than it is for other types of health care workers?**

   Nurses are positioned well to move easily and naturally into the management realm because of their clinical expertise, ability to facilitate interdisciplinary coordination, and knowledge of human and resource management. Nurses blend these skills to produce positive outcomes such as quality client care, workforce stability, organizational productivity, and effective cost control.

6. **Is case management a managerial role?**

   Case management involves the four elements of the management process: planning, organizing, coordinating or directing, and controlling. It is a care delivery approach designed to plan, organize, and coordinate care in order to control costs, increase quality outcomes, and enhance accessibility to appropriate and needed health care services.

Cultural Diversity

STUDY FOCUS

The growing appreciation for the global community has raised the awareness of cultural differences as well as the differing values in subcultures in local communities. For successful delivery of health care services, nurses must recognize the values of other cultures as they relate to health and take positive steps to recruit persons from other cultures to the nursing profession.

Cultural diversity is the variety and differences in the customs and practices of defined social groups. *Cultural competence* is providing care effectively to persons from a multiplicity of cultures. It is a dynamic and evolving process that embodies an evolution of knowing, respecting, and incorporating the values of others. Cultural competence involves the recognition of the importance of integrating persons with other values in the process of health care delivery. *Transcultural nursing* is a formal area of study and practice that focuses on cultural care, comparison of cultural variations, and the provision of culturally compassionate care.

The demographic makeup of the U.S. population in the areas of ethnicity and age are radically changing. Of the four major U.S. populations, the Hispanic and Asian-American/Pacific Islander groups are growing at a rapid rate (Freeman, 1997). Despite the rapidly changing demographic characteristics of the U.S. population, there is failure to obtain parity in positive health care outcomes for members of minority groups. Nurses are in a pivotal role to enact changes in effectively managing quality health care and managing resources to positively impact vulnerable populations in communities. Statistics show that 90% of the total registered nurse population is Caucasian. This is compared to 72% of the total U.S. population is Caucasian (U.S. Department of Health and Human Services, 1996). Recruitment efforts need to be aimed at attracting a diverse cultural mix of individuals into the nursing profession.

The predominant, Eurocentric, white majority has not carefully identified itself as having a valuable cultural heritage. A critical core concept in nursing is the awareness and recognition of cultural diversity. Nurses must be aware of their own Eurocentric concepts of patient autonomy, truth telling, and informed consent. Nurses must have an awareness of other cultures, but they do not have to agree with all the dominant beliefs of the culture. An important step in gaining cultural competence is recognizing one's own cultural beliefs.

To care effectively for culturally diverse clients, strategies must be employed to enhance cultural competence. Two strategies to enhance cultural competence include becoming cognitively aware of potential issues and building a repertoire of strategies to enhance cultural competence. Basic communication techniques such as how to properly address an individual and what a nod may mean can positively or adversely affect a nursing intervention. General guidelines for cultural competence include (a) nurses' awareness that their behavior may be perceived as abrupt when it is different from the client's cultural orientation, (b) being aware of the clients attitude toward suffering, (c) evaluating the fit of the treatment plan with the client's lifestyle, (d) anticipating that informed consent forms may be frightening, (e) recognizing the client's unfamiliarity with the nurse as professional staff and expectation that care will be delivered by a physician, and (f) realizing that Americans emphasize the clock, whereas other cultures may not.

It has been suggested that addressing cultural issues during the delivery of health care augments efforts at client compliance. The six areas often included in cultural assessments include communication, interpersonal space, social organization, sense of time, environmental control, and biological variation. Cultural beliefs about health and illness are learned and transmitted via cultural environments.

One culturally competent model of care was developed by Campinha-Bacote (1994). This model includes four components: (a) cultural awareness including sensitivity and biases, (b) cultural knowledge including worldviews and frameworks, (c) cultural skills including assessment tools, and (d) clinical encounters including exposure and practice. *Cultural awareness* is a deliberate cognitive process of becoming aware of and sensitive to the client's culture by becoming aware of one's own values and not imposing those values on others. *Cultural knowledge* is a process of obtaining information about the different world views of varying cultures. *Cultural skills* involve the process of learning how to do a cultural assessment. *Cultural encounter* is the process of engaging in cross-cultural interactions.

A trend in cultural awareness is the attracting of a culturally diverse workforce. The synergy of diverse viewpoints can improve health care knowledge and delivery of services. Strategies for success with cultural diversity in the workplace include respecting differences, exploring beyond the comfort zone, withholding judgment of others, and emphasizing the positive and practicing good communication. Diversity is the "consideration of socioeconomic class, gender, age, religious belief, sexual orientation, and physical disabilities, as well as rare and ethnicity" (AACN, 1997, p. 1). An issue that is becoming increasingly prevalent is that health illiteracy increases with age. Therefore, nursing interventions aimed at effective educational and communication strategies and materials to improve health care knowledge of the elderly are essential in the delivery of services.

LEARNING TOOLS

Group Activity: Characteristics of Selected Minorities

Purpose: To identify characteristics of selected minorities and to identify nursing strategies to produce positive health care outcomes for a select group.

Directions: Select three cultural groups in your geographical area that you would like to explore. Examples of dominant cultures within the United States include Mexican-American, African-American, Vietnamese-American, Chinese, Japanese, Cuban, and Puerto Rican.

On a sheet of paper list the major characteristics that you will research. Examples of major characteristics are listed below.

Cultural Group:

Language Spoken:

Predominant Religion:

Role of the Family:

Health care Practices:

Communication Patterns:

Risk Factors:

Compare and contrast the three cultural groups that you have researched. What characteristics are similar among the groups? What characteristics are different among the groups? How could you tailor interventions based on cultural beliefs to enhance positive health care outcomes?

Individual Activity: Giger and Davidhizar's Transcultural Assessment Model

Purpose: The transcultural assessment tool provides a comprehensive assessment format for culturally competent care. This assessment tool is a mechanism to evaluate cultural variables that influence health and illness behaviors.

Directions: Identify a client for whom you would like to complete a comprehensive cultural assessment. Use the tool below to identify cultural variables that will influence the nursing plan of care.

GIGER AND DAVIDHIZAR'S TRANSCULTURAL ASSESSMENT MODEL

Culturally Unique Individual

1. Place of birth
2. Cultural definition
   What is...
3. Race
   What is...
4. Length of time in country (if appropriate)

Communication

1. Voice quality
   A. Strong, resonant
   B. Soft
   C. Average
   D. Shrill
2. Pronunciation and enunciation
   A. Clear
   B. Slurred
   C. Dialect (geographical)
3. Use of silence
   A. Infrequent
   B. Often
   C. Length
      (1) Brief
      (2) Moderate
      (3) Long
      (4) Not observed
4. Use of nonverbal
   A. Hand movement
   B. Eye movement
   C. Entire body movement
   D. Kinesics (gestures, expression, or stances)
5. Touch
   A. Startles or withdraws when touched
   B. Accepts touch without difficulty
   C. Touches others without difficulty
6. Ask these and similar questions:
   A. How do you get your point across to others?
   B. Do you like communicating with friends, family, and acquaintances?
   C. When asked a question, do you usually respond (in words or body movement, or both)?
   D. If you have something important to discuss with your family, how would you approach them?

Space

1. Degree of comfort
   A. Moves when space invaded
   B. Does not move when space invaded
2. Distance in conversations
   A. 0 to 18 inches
   B. 18 inches to 3 feet
   C. 3 feet or more
3. Definition of space
   A. Describe degree of comfort with closeness when talking with or standing near others
   B. How do objects (e.g., furniture) in the environment affect your sense of space?
4. Ask these and similar questions:
   A. When you talk with family members, how close do you stand?
   B. When you communicate with coworkers and other acquaintances, how close do you stand?
   C. If a stranger touches you, how do you react or feel?
   D. If a loved one touches you, how do you react or feel?
   E. Are you comfortable with the distance between us now?

Social Organization

1. Normal state of health
   A. Poor
   B. Fair
   C. Good
   D. Excellent
2. Marital status
3. Number of children
4. Parents living or deceased?
5. Ask these and similar questions:
   A. How do you define social activities?
   B. What are some activities that you enjoy?
   C. What are your hobbies, or what do you do when you have free time?
   D. Do you believe in a Supreme Being?
   E. How do you worship that Supreme Being?
   F. What is your function (what do you do) in your family unit/system?
   G. What is your role in your family unit/system (father, mother, child, advisor)?

H. When you were a child, what or who influenced you most?
I. What is/was your relationship with your siblings and parents?
J. What does work mean to you?
K. Describe your past, present, and future jobs.
L. What are your political views?
M. How have your political views influenced your attitude toward health and illness?

Time

1. Orientation to time
   A. Past-oriented
   B. Present-oriented
   C. Future-oriented
2. View of time
   A. Social time
   B. Clock-oriented
3. Physiochemical reaction to time
   A. Sleeps at least 8 hours a night
   B. Goes to sleep and wakes on a consistent schedule
   C. Understands the importance of taking medication and other treatments on schedule
4. Ask these and similar questions:
   A. What kind of timepiece do you wear daily?
   B. If you have an appointment at 2 PM, what time is acceptable to arrive?
   C. If a nurse tells you that you will receive a medication in "about a half hour," realistically, how much time will you allow before calling the nurses' station?

Environmental Control

1. Locus-of-control
   A. Internal locus-of-control (believes that the power to affect change lies within)
   B. External locus-of-control (believes that fate, luck, and chance have a great deal to do with how things turn out)
2. Value orientation
   A. Believes in supernatural forces
   B. Relies on magic, witchcraft, and prayer to affect change
   C. Does not believe in supernatural forces
   D. Does not rely on magic, witchcraft, or prayer to affect change
3. Ask these and similar questions:
   A. How often do you have visitors at your home?
   B. Is it acceptable to you for visitors to drop in unexpectedly?
   C. Name some ways your parents or other persons treated your illnesses when you were a child.
   D. Have you or someone else in your immediate surroundings ever used a home remedy that made you sick?
   E. What home remedies have you used that worked? Will you use them in the future?
   F. What is your definition of "good health?"
   G. What is your definition of illness or "poor health?"

Biologic Variations

1. Conduct a complete physical assessment noting:
   A. Body structure (small, medium, or large frame)
   B. Skin color
   C. Unusual skin discolorations
   D. Hair color and distribution
   E. Other visible physical characteristics (e.g., keloids, chloasma)
   F. Weight
   G. Height
   H. Check lab work for variances in hemoglobin, hematocrit, and sickle phenomena if Black or Mediterranean
2. Ask these and similar questions:
   A. What diseases or illnesses are common in your family?
   B. Describe your family's typical behavior when a family member is ill.
   C. How do you respond when you are angry?
   D. Who (or what) usually helps you to cope during a difficult time?
   E. What foods do you and your family like to eat?
   F. Have you ever had any unusual cravings for:
      (1) White or red clay dirt?
      (2) Laundry starch?
   G. When you were a child what types of foods did you eat?
   H. What foods are family favorites or are considered traditional?

Nursing Assessment

1. Note whether the client has become culturally assimilated or observes own cultural practices.

2. Incorporate data into plan of nursing care:
   A. Encourage the client to discuss cultural differences; people from diverse cultures who hold different world views can enlighten nurses.
   B. Make efforts to accept and understand methods of communication.
   C. Respect the individual's personal need for space.
   D. Respect the rights of clients to honor and worship the Supreme Being of their choice.
   E. Identify a clerical or spiritual person to contact.
   F. Determine whether spiritual practices have implications for health, life, and well-being (e.g., Jehovah's Witnesses may refuse blood and blood derivatives; an Orthodox Jew may eat only kosher food high in sodium and may not drink milk when meat is served).
   G. Identify hobbies, especially when devising interventions for a short or extended convalescence or for rehabilitation.
   H. Honor time and value orientations and differences in these areas. Allay anxiety and apprehension if adherence to time is necessary.
   I. Provide privacy according to personal need and health status of the client (NOTE: the perception and reaction to pain may be culturally related).
   J. Note cultural health practices
      (1) Identify and encourage efficacious practices.
      (2) Identify and discourage dysfunctional practices.
      (3) Identify and determine whether neutral practices will have a long-term ill effect.
   K. Note food preferences
      (1) Make as many adjustments in diet as health status and long-term benefits will allow and that dietary department can provide.
      (2) Note dietary practices that may have serious implications for the client.

Giger, J.N. and R.E. Davidhizar (1995). *Transcultural Nursing: Assessment and Intervention* (2nd ed.). St. Louis: Mosby.

CASE STUDY

Juan, a 45-year-old migrant worker, presents to the clinic with fatigue, polydypsia, polyuria, and polyphagia. A translator is with Juan and tells you that he works in the fields from early morning to late evening picking produce. The health care provider orders laboratory tests and determines that Juan is diabetic. Juan is instructed on checking his blood glucose level, provided information in Spanish on diabetes, and instructed on medication administration. During the instruction Juan gets very upset when he is told to limit his intake of beverages with sugar. He tells the translator that he only has Koolaid in the fields because it is readily available and is provided by the employer.

Case Study Questions

1. How is your communication with the client influenced by the presence of a translator?
2. What cultural implications are apparent in this case study?
3. How will your nursing interventions be tailored to assist Juan in managing his diabetes?

LEARNING RESOURCES

Discussion Questions

1. How can nurses use information about various cultures to influence health care service delivery?
2. What is cultural diversity? What strategies can be employed to increase cultural diversity in the workforce?
3. What is the demographic makeup of the U.S. population? How does the demographic makeup in the U.S. compare to the demographics of the registered nursing population in the U.S.?
4. What does the "predominant, Eurocentric, white majority" mean? What are some Eurocentric concepts? How do these concepts affect the provision of nursing services?
5. What should a cultural assessment include?

Study Questions

True or False: Circle the correct answer.

T F 1. Cultural differences in ways of doing things and in beliefs about health and illness are learned and transmitted via cultural environments.

T F 2. Examples of cultural differences include eye contact norms, gender issues, touching and physical contact, and food practices.

T F 3. Japanese clients are usually given lower dosage levels of medications and have less tolerance for side effects.

T F 4. The term "Eurocentric" refers to valuing cultural diversity and being sensitive to cultural heritage.

T F 5. Minority groups obtain parity in positive health care outcomes when compared to the general overall health of the American people.

T F 6. Cultural competence is defined as an ongoing evolution of knowing, respecting, and incorporating the values of others.

Matching: Write the correct letter of the correct response in front of each term.

_____ 7. Cultural awareness

_____ 8. Cultural knowledge

_____ 9. Cultural skill

_____ 10. Cultural encounter

A. The process of seeking and obtaining an educational background about the different worldviews of various cultures

B. A process of directly engaging in cross-cultural interactions

C. The process of learning how to do a cultural assessment, allowing the nurse to identify an individual client's perceptions, beliefs, and practices

D. A deliberate and cognitive process of becoming aware of and sensitive to the client's culture by becoming aware of the influence of one's own cultural values and learning to avoid imposing them on others

REFERENCES

American Association of Colleges of Nursing (AACN). (1997). *Statement on diversity and equality of opportunity* {Online}. Available at www.aacn.nche.edu/Publications/positions/diverse.htm.

Freeman, H.P. (1997). Concerns of special populations in the national cancer program: The real impact of the reduction in cancer mortality research. In Meeting summary: *President's cancer panel* {Online}. Available at www.deainfo.nci.nih.gov/advisory/pcp/pcp0997/minutes.htm.

U.S. Department of Health and Human Services. (1996). *The registered nurse population*. Rockville, MD: Author.

SUPPLEMENTAL READINGS

Andrews, M.M. (1999). How to search for information on transcultural nursing and health subjects. *Journal of Transcultural Nursing, 10(1)*, 69-74.

Davidhizar, R., Havens, R., & Bechtel, G.A. (1999). Assessing culturally diverse pediatric clients. *Pediatric Nursing, 25(4)*, 371-376.

Hart, D. (1999). Assessing culture: Pediatric nurses' beliefs and self-reported practices. *Journal of Pediatric Nursing, 14(4)*, 255-262.

Martinez-Brawley, E.E. & Brawley, E.A. (1999). Diversity in a changing world: Cultural enrichment or social fragmentation? *Journal of Multicultural Social Work, 7*, 1-2, 19-36.

Narayan, M.C. (1997). Cultural assessment in home healthcare. *Home Healthcare Nurse, 15(10)*, 663-672.

Paniagua, H. (1999). Specialist nursing: Advanced nursing practice from a cross-cultural perspective. *British Journal of Nursing, 8(11)*, 724-729.

Riley-Eddins, E.A. (1999). The value of diversity. *Journal of Multicultural Nursing & Research, 5(1)*, 5.

ANSWERS TO TEXT STUDY QUESTIONS

Chapter 6—Cultural Diversity (p. 106)

1. **Why is cultural competence important for nursing?**

   Cultural competence is an ongoing process that involves expanding one's understanding of different cultures. As client advocates, nurses must be able to recognize, respect, and incorporate the values of other cultures in order to effectively deliver care. Knowing, respecting, and integrating the values and perspectives of others in care provision and organizational operations are needed to improve health services and to enhance the nursing profession.

2. **What are the components of cultural awareness?**

   Cultural awareness is the result of a purposeful, cognitive process involving a critical analysis of one's own cultural values and biases. Through deep reflection, one can become aware of and sensitive to other cultures without imposing one's own cultural expectations, attitudes, and behaviors. Without self-awareness and sensitivity, cultural competence cannot be achieved.

3. **How do you perform a cultural assessment?**

   Performing a cultural assessment provides an opportunity for the nurse to identify a client's perceptions, beliefs, and practices. According to Davidhizar, Bechtel, and Giger (1998), six cultural components to assess include communication, interpersonal space, social organization, sense of time, environmental control, and biologic variation. Other elements to assess include health care beliefs and practices, illness beliefs and customs, spiritual practices, and social structure features, including one's worldview. Nurses can use existing cultural assessment tools to assist in conducting a holistic data collection process.

4. **How does the nurse apply cultural competence in the workplace?**

   Nurses can use cultural competence to provide care to diverse clientele, to effectively lead and manage workgroups, and to enhance the nursing profession. Providing culturally competent care results in both client and staff satisfaction, and facilitates the success of the organization to recruit and maintain a culturally sensitive workforce. Nurses apply culturally competent strategies such as respect for differences, exploring beyond the comfort zone, withholding judgments of others, emphasizing the positive, and practicing good communication techniques to successfully lead and manage workgroups. A nursing profession that understands and respects other cultures will attract individuals to become members of its discipline, ultimately increasing the diversity and perspectives of the nurses providing care to the society.

Legal and Ethical Issues

STUDY FOCUS

Nurses are becoming increasingly aware of the extensive legal and ethical aspects to both nursing practice and nursing management. Professional autonomy indicates that the occupational group has control over its own practice. Individuals also have autonomy or the authority and accountability for their decisions and actions (Ballou, 1998). As the level of professional autonomy and responsibility increase, so does the level of accountability and liability (Aiken, 1994). Nurses often supervise others in daily activities. Supervision entails accountability for assigning tasks based on skill level, monitoring the tasks, and evaluating that the assigned tasks were performed adequately.

There are four types of law that must be dealt with in properly handling human resource decisions and actions. The four types of law include constitutional, statutory, case, and administrative. *Constitutional law* is law included in either the United States or state constitutions. *Statutory law* is law that has been enacted by the United States Congress, state legislatures, or local governing bodies, such as city councils or county governing boards. *Case law* is created when the courts, federal or state, render decisions and those decisions set precedents that need to be followed, at least in that court's jurisdiction. *Administrative law* includes those regulations promulgated and adopted by federal or state agencies to implement statutory law adopted by Congress or state legislatures.

Nurses have a duty of nonmalfeasance (to do no harm) to their clients. Harm may arise out of unintentional acts such as omission or intentional acts such as defamation or invasion of privacy. For malpractice to occur, four elements of negligence must be present. There must be a duty owed to the client, a breach of duty, proximate cause, and damages. Nurses and nurse managers are also responsible for reporting incompetent practices in the delivery of client care. Employers have the job of providing a safe and secure health care environment. The spectrum of legal and ethical consideration of nursing management includes the client, provider, and employer rights and obligations.

Employment discrimination laws were developed to prevent discrimination by employers of potential employees on the basis of race, sex, religion, national origin, physical disability, and age. Title VII of the U.S. Civil Rights Act of 1964 allows employers flexibility in limited situations to discriminate on the basis of *bona fide* occupational qualifications. Other employment-related laws include COBRA which focuses on health benefits to employees; ERISA which focuses on employee retirement benefits; and the Family and Medical Leave Act which provides flexibility in time off for medical reasons for the employee or family member. The Occupational Safety and Health Administration (OSHA) regulation is in place to monitor workplace environments. OSHA monitors workplaces through surprise inspections and levies heavy fines for noncompliance with safety standards.

Often, ethical issues arise from the distribution of scarce resources. *Professional loyalty* is the upholding of a client's interest over the professional's self-interest. Nurses are often faced with competing demands for loyalty in providing client care. Three aspects of an ethical practice environment include autonomy, trust, and communication. When malpractice and negligence occur, both the nurse and the employer are held liable under the doctrine of respondent superior. The employer is named as a defendant in a malpractice claim because employers are responsible for acts of employees.

There are several important terms in ethical decision making. The six cornerstones of ethical decision making include autonomy, beneficence, fidelity, justice, nonmalfeasance, and veracity. *Autonomy* is the client's right of self-determination and freedom of decision making. *Beneficence* is doing good for clients and providing benefit balanced against risk. *Fidelity* is being loyal and faithful to commitments and accountable for responsibility. *Justice* is being fair to all and giving equal treatment. *Nonmalfeasance* is doing no harm to clients. *Veracity* is telling the truth and not intentionally deceiving clients.

There are several ethical decision-making models used to solve problems. The MORAL model has five steps in ethical decision-making (Crisham, 1985). Step one is *massaging* the dilemma and defining the conflicts and interests. Step two is *outlining* options. Step three is *reviewing* criteria and resolving the dilemma. Step four is *affirming* a position and acting on the judgment. Step five is *looking* back to evaluate the effectiveness.

Individual values impact ethical decision-making. Values are beliefs or attitudes that are freely chosen and form a foundation for actions. Personal, professional, and organizational value sets have been identified. Berger, Seversen, and Chvatal (1991) reported that the most frequent ethical issues encountered by registered nurses was inadequate staffing, inadequate life support measures, inappropriate resource allocation, inappropriate discussion of patients, and irresponsible actions by coworkers. Inadequate staffing was the most frequently reported ethical problem.

Information published by the American Nurses Association in the pamphlet entitled *Nursing: A Social Policy Statement* outlines nursing's contract with society for safe and ethical practice and the ANA's Code of Ethics sets standards of conduct for nurses. Nurses constantly juggle ethical conflicts due to competing pressures from coworkers, clients, and the organization.

LEARNING TOOLS

Group Activity: Discussing Moral Issues in Nursing

Purpose: To gain a clear understanding of the ethical aspects of problem solving and to use an ethical decision-making model in problem resolution.

Directions: Discuss the ethical issues that affect nurses who work on the units to which you are assigned. Identify one ethical dilemma that the group would like to solve. Use the MORAL model described by Crisham (1985) for your discussions. Use the format below to guide the discussion.

Step one: Massage the dilemma and define the conflicts and interests.

____
____
____

Step two: Outline the potential options.

____
____
____

Step three: Review criteria for problem resolution and resolve the dilemma.

____
____
____

Step four: Affirm a position and act on the judgment.

____
____
____

Step five: Look back to evaluate the effectiveness of the decision.

____
____
____

CASE STUDY

Jo Ellen is a registered nurse on a 45-bed orthopedic unit in a community hospital. She works the 3-11 shift as a full-time employee. Jo Ellen is 32 years old and has three small children, ages 2, 4, and 7. She elects the 3-11 shift so that the children do not have to be in daycare. Her husband is an electrical engineer and is able to get home at 4:00 p.m. and Jo Ellen's mother watches the children for 1½ hours during the week. For the past six months the community hospital administration has enacted mandatory overtime for nurses because of a nurse shortage. Jo Ellen has been working approximately 2-3 mandatory shifts per week. She is very upset with working so much overtime and it is beginning to affect her family. She is so tired all the time trying to nap while the children play during the day.

Case Study Questions

1. What options does Jo Ellen have in relation to working the mandatory overtime?
2. What ethical decision-making concepts are important in Jo Ellen's predicament of mandatory overtime?
3. Use the MORAL model to solve Jo Ellen's ethical dilemma.

LEARNING RESOURCES

Group Activity: Identifying Current Ethical Issues

Purpose: To identify current ethical issues in nursing management and nursing practice settings.

Directions: Each individual selects one nurse manager and one registered nurse to interview. Ask each of the selected individuals the following question: What are the most pressing and difficult ethical issues you face in your work?

The group should meet at a set time and place and review the answers from the participants. What were the common ethical issues encountered by the managers and by the registered nurses? Were there any differences in the ethical issues between the two groups? How might you respond when faced with similar ethical issues?

Discussion Questions

1. What are ethical problems that have emerged around managed care organizations?
2. What are examples of reportable occurrences that registered nurses must manage?
3. What are the four types of laws that must be dealt with in properly handling human resource decisions?
4. What is the registered nurse's role in supervision and delegation of activities?
5. What is the doctrine of respondent superior?
6. What are the steps in the MORAL model? Identify an ethical dilemma in health care delivery and use the MORAL model to reach a decision strategy.

Study Questions

True or False: Circle the correct answer.

T F 1. Case law is the law included in either the United States or state constitutions.

T F 2. Administrative law includes those regulations promulgated and adopted by federal or state agencies to implement statutory law adopted by Congress or state legislatures.

T F 3. *Nursing: A Social Policy Statement* is a mandate for standards of conduct of nurses.

T F 4. Physicians govern the legal practice of nurses.

Matching: Write the letter of the correct response in front of each term.

_____ 5. Autonomy
_____ 6. Fidelity
_____ 7. Values
_____ 8. Veracity
_____ 9. Nonmalfeasance
_____ 10. Justice

A. Norm of telling the truth; not intentionally deceiving
B. Clients' right to self-determination and freedom of decision making
C. Strongly held beliefs that are thought to be freely chosen
D. Doing no harm to clients
E. Being loyal and faithful to commitments and accountable for responsibilities
F. Norm of being fair to all and giving equal treatment

REFERENCES

Aiken, T. (1994). *Legal, Ethical and Political Issues in Nursing*. Philadelphia: F.A. Davis.

Ballou, K.A. (1998). A concept analysis of autonomy. *Journal of Professional Nursing, 14(2)*, 102-110.

Berger, M., Seversen, A. & Chvatal, R. (1991). Ethical issues in nursing. *Western Journal of Nursing Research, 13(4)*, 514-521.

Crisham, P. (1985). Resolving ethical and moral dilemmas of nursing interventions. In M. Snyder (Ed.), *Independent nursing interventions* (pp. 25-43). New York: John Wiley & Sons.

SUPPLEMENTAL READINGS

Holt, J. & Long, T. (1999). Moral guidance, moral philosophy, and moral issues in practice. *Nursing Education Today, 19(3)*, 246-249.

Ketefian, S. (1999). Legal and ethical issues: Knowing good and doing good—is there a difference? *Journal of Professional Nursing, 15(1)*, 4.

Stearley, H. (1998). Fighting the good fight—legal issues and legislative update for nurses. *The Journal of Nurse Empowerment, 8(1)*, 23-28.

Trott, M.C. (1998). Legal issues for nurse managers. *Nursing Management, 29(6)*, 38-42.

Ventura, M.J. (1999). Legally speaking: When information must be revealed. *RN, 62(2)*, 61-2, 64, 75.

ANSWERS TO TEXT STUDY QUESTIONS

Chapter 7—Legal and Ethical Issues (p. 121)

1. **What governs the practice of nursing?**

   Nurse practice acts and professional regulation govern the practice of nursing. Nurse practice acts from each state govern the legal practice of nursing, including delegation and supervision, while professional standards and ethical codes regulate nursing practice. Licensure assures the public that individuals are properly prepared and competent to deliver nursing services.

2. **What types of laws affect the practice of nursing?**

   Constitutional, statutory, case, and administrative laws affect the practice of nursing. These societal laws affect personal liability related to clinical practice, delegation, and supervision. All nurses are accountable for their own acts, the use of knowledge and skills in the provision of care, and for delegation and supervision decisions.

3. **What happens when harm occurs?**

   Harm occurs when the actions of the nurse do not meet the standard of care and cause client injury. Harm can manifest itself as intentional or unintentional acts. Examples of harm include assault and battery, invasion of privacy, failure to follow hospital procedures, and failure to monitor. When harm occurs, the nurse may be subject to disciplinary action, legal repercussions, or professional sanctions.

4. **What laws govern organizational actions?**

   Employment laws govern organizational actions. Employment-related laws are designed to prevent employee discrimination, provide employee health and retirement benefits, and provide employees with a safe working environment. For example, Constitutional and federal laws prohibit discrimination based on employee sex, race, religion, national origin, disability, or age. COBRA laws govern employee health benefits, ERISA laws govern employee retirement benefits, and OHSA rules and regulations safeguard employee workplaces.

5. **What are the key ethical principles? How are they used?**

   There are six key ethical principles used in decision making: autonomy, beneficence, fidelity, justice, nonmalfeasance, and veracity. The six principles are used to guide decisions related to self-determination and freedom of decision making (autonomy), benefit versus risk (beneficence), loyalty and accountability (fidelity), fairness and equality (justice), doing no harm (nonmalfeasance), and truth telling (veracity).

6. **Why do ethical conflicts arise?**

   Ethical conflicts arise when clashes occur between ethical principles, professional values, and personal beliefs. As a result, individuals are forced to choose between competing and often divergent alternatives. Opposing beliefs and ideology may precipitate ethical conflicts requiring negotiation or mediation to resolve. In health care, ethical conflicts may arise from inadequate staffing, end-of-life issues, and resource allocation decisions.

Managing Time and Stress

STUDY FOCUS

Time is a valuable and elusive resource to manage. Time pressures create strong demands on nurses who must make difficult choices about accomplishing goals. Time management is accomplishing specific activities during the time available. Successful nurses set short-, medium-, and long-term goals and objectives for time management and implement well-thought-out strategies. Those who are successful at managing time say no, control interruptions, and delegate tasks. There are eight steps in the time management process. The steps include analyzing current time use with logs; analyzing the time logs to identify problems; conducting a self-assessment; setting goals and establishing priorities; developing action plans; implementing action plans via schedules, guides, or lists; developing techniques and solutions to improve time management problems; and following up on and evaluating time management patterns.

Time management is an important aspect of controlling and minimizing stress in personal and work-related activities. General strategies to control time include taking control of your calendar, planning ahead, simplifying documentation, and taming the telephone. The management of time and improvement of time managing strategies can increase goal accomplishment and decrease personal and professional stress.

Stress is part of a nurse's everyday work. Stress is a physical, psychosocial, or spiritual response to a stressful event called a stressor. *Job or occupational stress* is an uncomfortable sensation created by the demands of the job or work of the nurse. Nurses experience stress from many sources. Common stressors include clients who are dying or in pain, emergency treatments, demanding coworkers or clients, family commitments, situations in which personal safety is threatened, downsizing, and restructuring. A classic theory that describes stress and stressors is Selye's General Stress Theory. *Selye's theory of stress* describes stress as a nonspecific state in which each person responds individually to stressors. Most people respond in a fight-or-flight manner.

When stress is too great on the job, nurses may experience burnout. *Burnout* is a situation in which individuals, experiencing constant long-term stress, respond with emotional and/or physical exhaustion, decreased productivity, and overdepersonalization. New graduates can also experience stress caused by incongruity between their values of idealism and those of the actual work environment, called *reality shock*. New graduates often become disillusioned and decrease their productivity, change jobs, or return to school for a career change.

Coping effectively with stress and changes in the health care environment are essential for a satisfied, healthy, and productive employee. *Coping* is performing activities in an effort to adapt to the situation. *Cognitive appraisal* is an individual's assessment of the present stressful situation. *Stressors* can be internal or external to the nurse. *Internal stressors* can be the personal conflicts of balancing family, work, and social events. *External events* can include the work environment. Individuals react differently to stressors. Some may deny the existence of the stressors while others become optimistic that they will handle the stressful occurrence. *Personal hardiness*—a characteristic of commitment, control, and willingness to accept a challenge—has been postulated as being important in handling stress. Those nurses who are hardy are better able to manage their stress.

Hardy (1978) identified different types of role stress. *Role stress* occurs when individuals are unclear about their job obligations or they feel their obligations are impossible to meet. *Role strain* is a subjective feeling of distress arising from a response to outside forces. *Role ambiguity* is when role expectations are unclear to the nurse. *Role conflict* is experienced when role expectations are incompatible with each other. *Role incongruity* occurs when role expectations are incompatible with the professional values of the nurse. *Role overload* occurs when a nurse cannot possibly complete all assigned activities in the scheduled time frame. *Role underload* occurs when nurses with advanced training are not able to use their skills to the fullest extent.

Nurses must learn positive coping skills and adaptation strategies to function effectively in their personal and work lives. Individuals who cope effectively reduce their emotional distress, solve their problems, and maintain positive self-esteem. Nurses must carefully examine stressful situations and look out for their best interests. Coping strategies include spending time on recreational activities, creating a personal support network, being involved in a professional association, negotiating or resigning, walking away from problematic situations to reflect, complying when necessary, and modifying rules. Organizations that are attuned to employee well-being organize comprehensive stress management plans to benefit their workers. Strategies to improve well-being include physical activity, nutritional control, environmental control, and support groups.

Nurses have the responsibility for taking care of themselves and others to maximize health and wellness. When nurses become aware of staffing shortages, dangers to personal safety, poor interdepartmental relations, or inadequately designed team situations, they have an obligation to inform their managers of these problematic situations. Being part of a team that takes stressors and turns them into opportunities for innovations or learning boosts employee morale and satisfaction.

LEARNING TOOLS

Self-Assessment: Managing Time

Introduction: Organizing one's time is crucial. Time is a valuable asset. In the Western culture, we believe that time comes and goes; once it is gone, we cannot recover the moment. For individuals to effectively manage time, they must first determine what personal and professional goals are important for them to accomplish. This self-assessment includes three parts: identifying and prioritizing personal and professional goals, logging activities and amounts of time for each, and identifying and prioritizing activities.

Part I

Directions: Complete the following task: In the blank lines below, identify and prioritize by ranking five personal and professional goals for three time periods.

1-Year Personal Goals	5-Year Personal Goals	Lifetime Personal Goals
1. successfully complete my courses at LIU	1. become engaged → get married	1. Married c̄ children
2. graduate from LIU c̄ my BSN	2. maintain independence (apartment)	2. Own our home + more than one car
3. pass the NCLEX on my 1st try	3. own a car	3. Have an improved relationship c̄ my mother
4. maintain a part time job	4. travel	4. Travel
5. maintain my relationship c̄ my boyfriend	5. pregnant c̄ our first child	5. Enjoy my one + only life!

1-Year Professional Goals	5-Year Professional Goals	Lifetime Professional Goals
1. successfully complete my courses at LIU	1. keep thriving as an RN	1. Enjoy opportunities nursing will offer me.
2. graduate from LIU c̄ my BSN	2. establish myself at a facility	2. Be successful c̄ them.
3. pass the NCLEX on my 1st try	3. go back to school (MSN)	3. Have excellent critical thinking skills
4. If not - take Kaplan	4. Successfully complete my MSN courses	4. Experience different areas of nursing
5. Pass NCLEX on my 2nd try.	5. graduate	5. Be a GOOD nurse!

The task of identifying and prioritizing your personal and professional goals is very time consuming and difficult, but essential for you to manage your time effectively. Annually you should revisit your list and update as well as congratulate yourself on accomplishments.

Part II

Directions: For a 24-hour period write down all activities that you complete as well as the time you engaged in the activity in a small notebook. After you have made a 24-hour record, determine the number of minutes engaged in each activity. A sample log is illustrated below.

Time Started	Time Completed	Activity	Total Time in Minutes
12:00 am	8:45 am	Sleep	525
8:46 am	9:05 am	wash up + listen to music	19
9:06 am	11:30 am	study psych.	144
11:31 am	11:50 am	spoke to boyfriend on phone	19
11:51 am	12:15 pm	cook	14
12:15 pm	12:40 pm	eat	25
12:41 pm	1:45 pm	shower + dress for work	64
1:46 pm	2:20 pm	travel on subway to work	24
2:21 pm	7:25 pm	do work + sneak to study psych. notes	304
7:26 pm	8:05 pm	travel on subway to home	39
8:06 pm	8:30 pm	eat dinner, change clothes, wash up	24
8:31 pm	9:00 pm	slept	29
9:01 pm	9:10 pm	spoke to boyfriend on phone	9
9:11 pm	9:40 pm	slept	29
9:41 pm	1:30 am	studied for psych. exam	229

This activity is useful in at least three ways. First, it identifies any time robbers such as interruptions, unproductive meetings, telephone solicitations, unorganized activities, and time wasters that may be filling your day. Secondly, it shows you what activities you chose to spend your time doing. That way you can compare these activities to your personal and professional goals to see if they are congruent, or if you need to reprioritize your activities. Finally, it shows you your style of time management. Are you managing a crisis constantly? Are you spending all of your time in professional activities? How much personal time do you have?

Part III

Directions: Identify those personal and professional activities that are most important to you and prioritize them. This is the easy task because you have already established your goals. Now, make a daily or weekly list of activities that you need to accomplish and check them off as they are completed. This checklist should be a tool and should not become the center of time management. Below is an example of a checklist. You may rank your activities according to their priority or star those that are most critical to complete first.

This activity helps to organize your daily and weekly workload into a manageable list.

	Activities to Accomplish	Date to Be Completed	Check when Completed
1.	maintain my health		
2.	maintain my home life.		
3.	do my best at school.		
4.	get adequate rest.		
5.	graduate school		
6.	pass my NCLEX		
7.	get a good job.		
8.	thrive as an RN		
9.	get married		
10.	have children.		

Self-Assessment Stress Test

Purpose: To assess your level of stress.

Directions: Check each event that you have experienced during the past 12 months.

Event	Value	Score
Death of spouse	100	_____
Divorce	73	_____
Marital separation	65	_____
Jail term	63	_____
Death of close family friend	63	_____
Personal injury or illness	53	_____
Marriage	50	_____
Fired from work	47	_____
Marital reconciliation	45	_____
Retirement	45	_____
Change in family member's health	44	_____
Pregnancy	40	_____
Sex difficulties	39	_____
Addition to family	39	_____
Business readjustment	39	_____
Change in financial status	38	_____
Death of close friend	37	_____
Change to different line of work	36	_____
Change in number of marital arguments	35	_____
Mortgage or loan over $100,000	31	_____
Foreclosure of mortgage or loan	30	_____
Change in work responsibilities	29	_____
Son or daughter leaving home	29	_____
Trouble with in-laws	29	_____
Outstanding personal achievement	28	_____
Spouse begins or stops work	26	_____
Starting or finishing school	26	_____
Change in living conditions	25	_____
Revision of personal habits	24	_____
Trouble with boss	23	_____
Change in work hours conditions	20	_____
Change in residence	20	_____
Change in schools	20	_____
Change in recreational habits	19	_____
Change in church activities	19	_____
Change in social activities	18	_____
Mortgage or loan under $100,000	17	_____
Change in sleeping habits	16	_____
Change in number of family gatherings	15	_____
Change in eating habits	15	_____
Vacation	13	_____
Christmas season	12	_____
Minor violations	11	_____
	Total Points	_____

Scoring: Add up your score of stress related events which occurred during the last 12 months. If your score falls at 150 points or less you're fairly safe from developing a stress-related illness. If your score falls between 151-299 you have a 50% chance of developing a stress-related illness and if your score is 300 or more you have an 80% chance of developing a stress-related illness.

Reprinted by permission of the publisher from "The Social Readjustment Rating Scale," Holmes, T.H. & Rahe, R.H., *Journal of Psychosomatic Research*, vol. 11, pp. 213-218. Copyright 1967 by Elsevier Science Inc.

CASE STUDY

Kelsey, a clinical nurse on a 18-bed protective care unit in a community hospital in Rock Springs, Wyoming, has worked for the hospital for 20 years. Kelsey has observed many changes at the hospital, but lately there are several changes occurring at once with restructuring, quality improvement processes, downsizing, and the addition of UAPs. Kelsey has been feeling physically exhausted and depersonalized, and her productivity is declining. Kelsey feels helpless and would like all the changes to stop, so that she could just provide good individualized client care. Lately, coworkers have noticed that Kelsey does the minimum possible to get by and leaves promptly at the stroke of 3:00 p.m. when her shift ends.

Case Study Questions

1. What syndrome is Kelsey experiencing?
2. What is causing her to feel helpless and to begin to decompensate?
3. What can Kelsey do now to help herself function effectively when providing client care?

LEARNING RESOURCES

Discussion Questions

1. What are effective coping strategies for nurses to use in order to stay healthy and deliver optimal client care?
2. What is occupational or job stress? What causes job stress? How can nurses work effectively when experiencing job stress?
3. What is Selye's General Stress Theory? Describe how this theory is applicable to nursing.
4. What is the difference between reality shock and burnout? Describe and give an example of each.
5. How can nurses be proactive and use stress to their benefit? Give an example.

Study Questions

Matching: Write the letter of the correct response in front of each term.

_____ 1. Stress
_____ 2. Stressor
_____ 3. Burnout
_____ 4. Reality shock
_____ 5. Role incongruity
_____ 6. Role ambiguity
_____ 7. Hardiness
_____ 8. Role overload
_____ 9. Role underload
_____10. Role strain

A. Occurs when nurses with advanced training are not able to use their skills to the fullest
B. When a nurse cannot possibly complete all assigned activities in the scheduled time frame
C. When role expectations are incompatible with the professional values of the nurse
D. When role expectations are unclear to the nurse
E. Subjective feeling of distress arising from responses to outside forces
F. New graduates' experience of incongruity in their values of idealism in the work environment
G. Long-term success resulting in exhaustion or decreased productivity
H. Characteristics of commitment, control, and willingness to accept a challenge
I. A stressful event
J. A physical, social, or spiritual response to an event

REFERENCE

Hardy, M.E. (1978). Role stress and role strain. In M.E. Hardy & M.E. Conway (Eds.), *Role Theory: Perspectives for Health Professionals* (2nd Ed.). Norwalk, CT: Appleton-Century-Crofts.

SUPPLEMENTAL READINGS

Charnley, E. (1999). Occupational stress in the newly qualified staff nurse. *Nursing Stanford, 13(29)*, 33-36.

Davidson, J. (1998). How to create more time and space in your life. *Vital Speeches of the Day, 64(11)*, 327-332.

Davidhizar, R., Newman, J., Giger, V. & Poole, L. (1998). Time-bound madness. *The Health Care Manager, 17(2)*, 28-35.

Merry, M. & Singer, D. (1994). Healing the healers. *Healthcare Forum Journal, 37(6)*, 37-41.

Stetson, B. (1997). Holistic health stress management program. *Journal of Holistic Nursing, 15(2)*, 143-157.

VanGerpen, R. (1999). Nurses need time for recreation, rest, and reflection. *Oncology Nursing Society News, 14(1)*, 1, 4-5.

Wolff, P. & Ratner, P.A. (1999). Stress, social support, and sense of coherence. *Western Journal of Nursing Research, 21(2)*, 182-197.

ANSWERS TO TEXT STUDY QUESTIONS

Chapter 8—Time and Stress (p. 137)

1. **Why is self-management so important to time management?**

   Self-management allows an individual to control the time management process. Individuals who develop their own time management strategies are empowered to select approaches that will maximize available resources to achieve personal and professional commitments and goals. Selecting specific, measurable, and realistic activities that are personally relevant increases the likelihood that effective and efficient time management strategies will be implemented and actualized.

2. **What strategies of time management work best for nurses?**

   Time management strategies that work best for nurses include analyzing the workday and prioritizing the workload. Depending on the individual situation, available resources, and safety concerns, different strategies may be selected and implemented. Time may be successfully managed through the use of checklists; delegation; planning ahead; and by dividing large projects or tasks into smaller, more manageable undertakings. Time management strategies may differ depending on the practice setting. For example, in home health care, Sherry (1996) identified six time management strategies: take control of your calendar, minimize time spent in office, tame the telephone, simplify documentation, plan ahead, and save time for others.

3. **What sources of stress do you find to be the most important influences in your life and work?**

   Nurses face many sources of stress in their personal and professional lives. The sources of stress that are the most influential affect your ability to control a given situation or circumstance. Sources of personal stress may include concerns related to childcare, fatigue, or financial obligations. Workplace stresses may include issues related to role expectations, interpersonal communication, environment, patient care situations, or knowledge deficits.

4. **What coping strategies are most helpful for stress reduction? Why are they helpful?**

   An individual's personality characteristics, perceptions of the external environment, and past experiences with similar stressors determine which coping mechanisms are selected as most useful. Coping mechanisms are used to maintain or regain equilibrium in order to adjust to stressful situations. Effective coping mechanisms reduce emotional distress, enhance problem resolution, and facilitate self-esteem. Examples of coping strategies include humor, complying, resigning, using a support network, spending time with hobbies, and using relaxation techniques.

5. **To what extent should employers pay for stress management programs for nurses?**

   Human resources are the largest fiscal expenditure for organizations. Work-related stress can lead to job dissatisfaction, poor performance, and high turnover rates. High turnover rates result in increased personnel costs secondary to new employee recruitment and orientation. Employee-oriented organizations establish stress management programs to minimize occupational stress so as to foster job satisfaction, productivity, and retention.

6. **Why should nurses manage their own stress?**

   The health care environment is stressful, with high client acuity levels, inadequate staffing, specialty care requirements, ethical dilemmas, and dangerous situations that jeopardize individual safety. In addition, each professional nurse has her or his own personal stressors. Taking steps to proactively manage and minimize the stress in your personal and professional lives will enhance your level of productivity and satisfaction.

7. **Why should nurses promote reality shock support for new graduates?**

   New graduates often experience personal and professional stressors as they make the transition from student to professional practitioner. Novice nurses in their first year of professional practice may experience disillusionment, dismay, and incongruence with organizational values. Experienced nurses can assist, mentor, and council new graduates to recognize stressors and to develop effective stress management strategies.

8. **What can nurses do to manage stress in work teams?**

   Identification of stressors, effective communication, conflict resolution, and group support minimize stress in work teams. As the work team becomes more knowledgeable about stressors, collaboration occurs to design effective strategies to reduce stress in the work environment.

Motivation

STUDY FOCUS

The United States is transitioning from the industrial age to an information age. Knowledgeable workers, lateral organizations, and an interdisciplinary focus characterize the nature of work required in an information age. Integration and motivation of employees in highly specialized environments require creativity and blending of leadership, management, and motivation.

Motivation is a complex process requiring strong leadership and management skills to creatively enhance employee productivity. Nurse managers of health care organizations are faced with trying to increase employee productivity while maintaining or decreasing labor costs. Motivation is the perception of the person toward a goal, which energizes them to act. An activity is the basic unit of behavior. Individuals perform activities based on their motives or needs, what they desire or want. Nurse managers are challenged to motivate employees to work in a way that achieves organizational goals expeditiously. Energizing, facilitating, and maintaining high levels of employee productivity is often problematic.

Traditionally, managers of bureaucratic organizations use direct supervision to control employees; whereas managers using a human relations approach in decentralized organizations employ the methods of participation and cooperation. Many motivational models have been developed to help guide managers in motivating employees to maximum productivity. The Needs Satisfaction Model states that there is a felt need followed by an activity or behavioral response. Then a process results to decrease frustration and meet individual needs. Individual needs arise from both internal and external motivating forces. Internal motivation is a personal desire to achieve and accomplish. On the other hand, external motivation is a stimulus external to an individual that generates an incentive to complete an activity.

Maslow's Hierarchy of Needs Theory is based on levels of human needs starting with basic needs and ending with self-actualization. Maslow's hierarchy includes five levels —physiological drives, safety and security needs, belonging needs, esteem and ego needs, and self-actualization. Maslow's work was refined by Alderfer who collapsed the five levels to three which include existence, relatedness, and growth needs.

Herzberg's Motivation-Hygiene Theory describes two categories of needs, hygiene or maintenance factors and motivators. *Hygiene or maintenance factors* are security, status, money, working conditions, interpersonal relations, supervision, and policies and administration. *Motivators* include the need for growth and development, advancement, increased responsibility, challenging work, recognition, and achievement. Motivators encourage superior performance while hygiene factors maintain satisfaction.

McClelland's theory describes three basic needs: achievement, power, and affiliation. McClelland's theory lends itself to self-assessment. Nursing leaders were found to have no need to moderately high levels of need for power, low levels of affiliation needs, high levels of self-control needs, and minimal achievement motivation.

Expectancy theories, including Vroom's, examine the attractiveness of an outcome, a valence, and the likelihood that the outcome will occur. In these theories, employees assess the value of an outcome and the degree to which individuals perceive that they can attain the reward. Then they decide whether they will expend the energy to perform the activity.

Job characteristics theory examines the job, the individual, and the outcome. Core job dimensions of the theory include task identity, task significance, skill variety, and autonomy and feedback. The core job dimensions interact with three critical psychological states—the meaningfulness of the work, responsibility for outcomes, and the actual result of the work. The outcomes may improve productivity, enhance quality, decrease turnover and absenteeism, and improve personal and professional job satisfaction.

McGregor published *theory X and theory Y*. Theory X's basic assumptions are that employees are lazy and nonproductive and require close supervision. It portrays employees as resistant to autonomy and unable to assume responsibility. In contrast, theory Y's basic assumptions are that employees enjoy autonomy and need only guidance as opposed to supervision. Employees are depicted as creative, self-directed individuals who embrace responsibility and autonomy.

The classic *Hawthorne studies* were conducted in 1924 at the Hawthorne plant of Western Electric. The studies examined the motivation and productivity of assembly line workers. Several variables—including improving lighting, scheduling breaks, providing lunches, and shortening work hours—were studied with control and experimental groups. To the researchers' surprise, all the variables had a significant positive impact upon employee productivity. Even after all the variables were withdrawn productivity climbed. Study outcomes showed that interpersonal relationships were also a significant factor in motivating employees.

Organizational commitment is the intensity of an individual's identification with and involvement in the employing organization. Employee involvement is their participation in decision making. Employees are key assets in an information society. Managers must use creative strategies to maximize the human talents and achieve high levels of productivity in their organizations.

Nurses are motivated by personal, professional, and economic recognition. Verbal feedback has been identified as the most meaningful form of recognition for nurses. Five types of recognition are verbal feedback, written feedback, public acknowledgment, advancement and growth opportunities, and compensation. Other major influences motivating nurses are job enjoyment, quality care, caring by their superior/boss, adequate staffing, and a safe work environment. Nurses are compensated economically via base, variable, and indirect pay. *Base pay* is salary for work performed; variable pay includes bonuses and incentive pay; and indirect pay includes benefits such as health insurance, sick time, and vacation pay. Many employees view pay as an entitlement. It does not motivate them, but it does prevent dissatisfaction when adequate.

Managers must structure environments to enhance productivity. Demotivation often occurs when there are organizational restructuring, redesign, downsizing, increased use of temporary workers, and shifts in jobs. Managers are challenged to motivate employees in turbulent environments. Elements that affect motivation include goals, expectations, feedback, reinforcement, responsibility, trust, and rewards. Motivating techniques include using formal rewards, tailoring rewards to the employee, and providing immediate feedback. The current trends in nursing are to use formal recognition by designating heroes and heroines and reframing responsibilities. Demotivation is low morale in organizations.

LEARNING TOOLS

Role Play: Motivating Subordinates to Improve Productivity

Character One = Jo Ellen is the nurse manager of a neurorespiratory unit of a medium-sized hospital in Beaumont, Texas. Jo Ellen believes in rewarding staff for superior performance and tailors reward based on individual accomplishments.
Character Two = Bob is an RN who was hired ten years ago and has been doing an adequate, but not exemplary job.
Character Three = Jon is an RN who was hired five years ago and who consistently exhibits superior performance in client care.
Character Four = Jane is an RN who was hired one year ago and consistently performs well.

• • • • •

Jo Ellen is preparing annual reviews (performance appraisals) on all of her employees. She knows that Jon, Bob, and Jane are best friends and share information with each other. Jo Ellen wants to reward Jon and Jane for their exemplary performance, but does not want Bob disgruntled. Jo Ellen decides to give special merit pay to Jon and award him the neurological nurse of the year because he consistently performs outstandingly. Jo Ellen also puts Jane's name in for the hospital's professional nurse of the year award and sends her to a national neurosurgical nursing convention in California. One morning, Jo Ellen enters the neurorespiratory unit to see Jane, Bob, and Jon arguing loudly in the conference room. Upon entering the conference room, Bob aggressively approaches Jo Ellen and demands an explanation for her poor choices as a manager. Bob demands to know why his ten years of loyal service were not recognized. What should Jo Ellen do?

Role-Play Questions

1. What should Jo Ellen say? Should she give Bob a reward?
2. What strategies can be used to motivate Bob to work harder?
3. How can Jo Ellen manage the situation to empower all three individuals?

Role-Play Worksheet

Characters	Student Assigned
Jo Ellen, the nurse manager	______
Bob, RN of 10 years	______
Jon, RN of 5 years	______
Jane, RN of 1 year	______

Which character have you been assigned?

What are your character's goals in this situation?

How can the other characters assist you in achieving your goals?

What might the other characters do to hinder you in achieving your goals?

What strategies and probes do you plan to use in this situation?

CASE STUDY

Jackie is a charge nurse on the 11-7 shift at Middleville Hospital in Little Rock, Arkansas. Jackie's leadership style includes directing employees to accomplish tasks. She feels that the nurse's aides, licensed practical nurses (LPN), and orderlies are lazy and do only what they are required to do. Jackie requires them to report to her any client changes, large or small, because she feels they cannot handle responsibility. Jackie has developed detailed, step-by-step procedures for her staff to follow to prevent mistakes.

Case Study Questions

1. What motivational theory is Jackie practicing from?
2. What are the characteristics of this theory?
3. Is this an effective theory to practice leadership behaviors?
4. What motivational theory might you use when assigned the job of charge nurse?

LEARNING RESOURCES

Discussion Questions

1. What types of rewards motivate nurses to improve productivity?
2. What did the Hawthorne studies show? Why were the Hawthorne studies' results important to managers?
3. What is the difference between internal and external motivation? How can a nurse manager capitalize on these?
4. What is the difference between the needs satisfaction model and Vroom's theory?
5. How can you apply Maslow's hierarchy of needs theory to nursing management?
6. In an information age, what is the nature of the work needed in health care organizations? How does the nature of work differ from the industrial age to the information age?
7. What is demotivation and what factors create this problem in organizations?

Study Questions

Matching: Write the letter of the correct response in front of each term.

_____ 1. Motivation
_____ 2. Motives
_____ 3. External motivation
_____ 4. Variable pay
_____ 5. Activity
_____ 6. Internal motivation
_____ 7. Indirect pay
_____ 8. Base pay
_____ 9. Vroom's theory
_____ 10. McClelland's theory

A. A unit of human behavior
B. Benefits like sick and vacation time
C. Salary received for work completed
D. Gain sharing, bonuses, and incentive pay
E. Identifies people's basic needs
F. Represents valence, instrumentality, and expectancy
G. Energizing and eliciting human activity
H. Wants, desires, and drives
I. Individuals who provide incentives for activity
J. Accomplishments arising from within the individual

True or False: Circle the correct answer.

T F 1. Demotivation is rewarding employees for a job well done.

T F 2. Knowledge workers, lateral organizations, and an interdisciplinary focus characterize the information age.

T F 3. Organizational commitment is a strong involvement and identification with the employing organization.

T F 4. The reward that has been found to be most effective in increasing employee productivity is pay.

T F 5. Herzberg's Motivation-Hygiene Theory describes three basic needs: achievement, power, and affiliation.

SUPPLEMENTAL READINGS

Breisch, L.R. (1999). Motivate! *Nursing Management, 30(3)*, 27-30.

Edgar, L. (1999). Nurses' motivation and its relationship to the characteristics of nursing care delivery systems: A test of the Job Characteristics Model. *Canadian Journal of Nursing Leadership, 12(1)*, 14-21.

Janssen, P.P., de Jonge, J. & Bakker, A.B. (1999). Specific determinants of intrinsic work motivation, burnout and turnover intentions: A study among nurses. *Journal of Advanced Nursing, 29(6)*, 1360-1369.

Kelley, R. & Caplan, J. (1993). How Bell Labs creates star performers. *Harvard Business Review, 71(4)*, 128-139.

Keyes, M. (1994). Recognition and reward: A unit-based program. *Nursing Management, 25(2)*, 52-54.

Salvatore-Magalhaes, J. (1999). Remember where you came from. *Nursing Management, 30(5)*, 29-30.

Tye, J. (1997). Never fear, never quit. *Nursing Management, 28(7)*, 38-40.

ANSWERS TO TEXT STUDY QUESTIONS

Chapter 9—Motivation (p. 163)

1. **How do you stay motivated to love nursing for the rest of your life?**

   It is important for nurses to be cognizant of the factors that provide them internal and external motivation. Ask yourself which values, beliefs, and assumptions motivate you to love nursing? How have they changed? Will the same factors motivate you in the future? What impact will career advancement, increased responsibility, and work challenges have on your motivation?

2. **Does loving nursing guarantee quality care?**

   While loving nursing cannot guarantee quality care, the nurse's motivation is a powerful influence on the provision of quality care. The love of nursing may serve as an internal force that motivates nurses to provide excellent care, which in turn may generate external reinforcement from positive patient outcomes and professional satisfaction.

3. **What is the motivation to enter nursing as a career? Is this changing?**

   Individuals enter nursing for a variety of reasons. Some individuals are motivated by the need for recognition, acknowledgment, status, or economic compensation, while others are motivated by the need for autonomy, a sense of doing important work, helping others, the need for competence, or self actualization. Motivation to enter nursing as a career may change depending on expanded roles, educational requirements, professional recognition, societal contribution, and competitive salaries.

4. **What is the comparison of real-world nursing practice to what motivation theories say?**

   Many motivation theories can be applied to real-world nursing practice. For example, nurses use the Need Satisfaction Model in the provision of care, as well as Maslow's Hierarchy of Needs theory to formulate effective teaching strategies. Herzberg's Motivation-Hygiene theory fits well in describing job satisfaction and dissatisfaction.

   Real-world nursing practice is affected by challenging work, collegial relationships, and professional/societal recognition. In order to ascend the self-actualization hierarchy, nurses must perceive safe working conditions, administrative support, and financial security.

5. **What positive incentives are most important to nurses? To you personally?**

   Positive incentives vary depending on the needs of the individual nurse. The love of the work itself is often a significant motivator for nurses. Positive incentives may include providing quality client care, client advocacy, professional acknowledgment, and a challenging work environment. What professional, personal, and financial incentives are important to you?

6. **What are the elements of a motivating environment?**

   Elements of a motivating environment include explicit goals, clear expectations, direct feedback and reinforcement, elimination of threats, individual responsibility, rewards, and trust. The nurse leader's job is to create an environment that fosters motivation by identifying what nurses need to succeed, to be satisfied, and to feel what they do is an important service to clients.

7. **Is it manipulative or Machiavellian to deliberately plan and implement rewards and incentives to get other people to reform? Do you ever do this?**

   The art of leading and managing groups of professional nurses requires creative, interesting, and innovative ways to make people feel good about what they are doing. While the rewards and incentives can be viewed as manipulative, it is a mutually beneficial relationship in which recognition is provided in exchange for quality performance. Personal, professional, and economic rewards have been shown to be powerful motivators in nursing.

8. **Under cost-containment pressures, what is the effect on nurses of relying on recognition as the organizational motivation strategy?**

   Cost-containment pressures may create dissatisfaction in nurses who rely on economic rewards as an entitlement or as a motivator to perform. Productivity may decrease while perceptions of betrayal and cynicism increase. Nurse leaders may need to develop and implement personal and professional recognition programs to compensate for the loss of economic rewards.

Power and Conflict

STUDY FOCUS

Power gives us control and freedom. *Power* is the ability to influence another's actions in order to attain a scarce resource. *Empowerment* is giving responsibility and accountability to individuals to complete tasks. There is personal and professional power. *Personal power* is the extent to which individuals can influence events through their own personal effort, while *professional power* is influence that results from doing a good job and interacting with colleagues.

The eight mechanisms people use to gain power include assertiveness, ingratiation, rationality, sanctions, exchange, upward appeal, blocking, and coalitions. *Assertiveness* is standing up for your rights without infringing on others' rights. *Ingratiation* is praising someone for a job well done in hopes of gaining recognition for your support. *Rationality* is the logical presentation of ideas. *Sanctions* include the use of threats and negative activities to gain a desired response. *Exchanges* are trades for services or goods in which both parties receive something desired. *Upward appeals* involve the act of seeking opinion of a higher authority about a decision. *Blocking* is stopping someone's activities or progress by threatening them, ignoring them, or physically interfering with their progress. *Coalitions* are the banding together of individuals for the purpose of a single voice.

Raven and French identify five sources of power. *Reward power* is the use of praise, pay, promotions, or advancements. *Coercive power* is the use of force such as threatening to fire an individual or to discipline them. *Expert power* is based on knowledge, competence, and skill. *Referent power* is based on a person's interpersonal appeal, charisma, and image. *Legitimate power* is based on the job title or position a person holds. Other sources of power include connection, a network of powerful people or information sources, and informational power, the control of special information.

In organizations, formal power is attained through position. Nurse managers must use power to be effective in leading the staff in care delivery. The four sources of organizational power include structural position, personal characteristics, expertise, and opportunity. Structural position is positional power and includes centrality, control of uncertainty, and control over resources. Individuals accrue power by the centrality of their work to the organization's mission and the visibility and discretion associated with their job. Personal characteristics incorporate the culture, values, and mix.

To be powerful, one must be able to access support, information, and resources, and must be aware of opportunities to seize advancement or achievements. Those who use power positively resolve conflicts with creativity, innovation, and novelty, whereas those who use power ineffectively create barriers, decrease efficiency, and encourage distrust and uncomfortable work environments. Strategies to gain and maintain power include gaining access to information, controlling resources, accessing key decision makers, and networking with powerful individuals.

Power moments refer to those occasions when one individual interferes with another's power. Strategies that may be used during power moments include fights, which engage two or more people in a struggle for the same resource; negotiation, where two or more people respectfully discuss the situation and come to an agreement; and collaboration, where two or more individuals cooperate to determine a solution. Multiple power sources need to be used to avoid diminished power resources. Political strategies include forming coalitions, bargaining, lobbying, posturing or bluffing, and increasing visibility.

Empowering others promotes excellence and motivates others. Empowerment, a method to improve productivity, lower costs, and raise customer satisfaction is an important strategy for organizational productivity. Two forms of empowerment initiatives are the relational and motivational approach. In the relational approach, performance is improved through decentralization. The motivational approach focuses on open communication and inspirational goal setting. Increasing empowerment has been linked to effective performance.

Conflict is natural and can be a useful growth experience for individuals. Conflict arises between two or more individuals from a perceived threat to their wants, needs, feelings, behaviors, or attitudes. Organizational conflict arises from competition for the limited available resources in an organization. Job conflict is the struggle between individual and organizational goals. Conflict occurs because of discord between one individual's values, philosophies, and beliefs and those of other individuals. When conflict is handled positively, there can be personal or professional growth; improved relationships; and increased productivity, creativity, and satisfaction. When it is handled poorly, fear, retaliation, anger, and hostility are the result.

Conflict can be categorized three ways—intrapersonal, interpersonal, and intergroup. Intrapersonal conflict arises within an individual from two competing demands or ideas. *Interpersonal conflict* is the battle between two or more individuals arising from miscommunication or differences in values. *Intergroup conflict* is the result of struggles between two or more groups. Conflict can be either competitive, when the individuals strive to win, or it may be disruptive, when the intent is to defeat, eliminate, or harm the opponent.

Pondy (1967) has identified five stages of conflict. The first stage is antecedent conditions, which are the conditions that begin stirring the pot of discontent. Examples could include the competition for resources, differing goals, or a lack of individual responsibility. The second stage, perceived conflict, emerges, and emotions become charged. During the third stage, an individual has a felt conflict and expresses these emotions. The individual initiates behavior to correct or alleviate the felt conflict either by negatively talking about the other individuals, by initiating actions to correct the situation, or by removing himself from the uncomfortable environment. Manifest behavior occurs in the fourth stage when the individual acts and either resolves or suppresses the conflict. The fifth and final stage, aftermath to the conflict, occurs when there is an effect, either resolution to the conflict or a cyclic process in which increasing antecedent behaviors take place.

There are three strategies that can be used to resolve organizational conflicts: bargaining; using rules, procedures, and administrative control; and using a system integrator. Nurses can experience conflict in the form of role overload, in which they are required to do the work of other health care disciplines; in role ambiguity, in which the nurses' responsibilities and duties expand without a job description change; or role stress, where a nurse's boss has one idea about the job and the nurse has a different perception.

Effectively managing conflict is essential for positive work groups. There are three frameworks for resolving conflict: defensive, compromise, and creative. The defensive mode leaves individuals feeling both losses and wins. Strategies for defensively addressing conflict are separating the competing parties, suppressing conflict, restricting the conflict, smoothing over the conflict through change, and avoiding the conflict. A compromise mode solves conflict through negotiation until a mutually acceptable solution is reached in which each party receives something and forfeits something. The creative problem-solving mode is the best possible scenario, where all parties gain and do not feel a loss. In creative conflict resolution, a five-step process is used: initiating discussion at a set time in private, understanding and respecting differences, empathizing with each party, engaging in an assertive discussion, and agreeing on a solution.

Conflict resolution techniques include avoiding, withholding, smoothing over, accommodating, forcing, competing, compromising, confronting, collaborating, bargaining, and problem solving. Outcomes for conflict resolution include win-win, win-lose, and lose-lose. Win-lose is when one party wins without concern about the other. Win-win occurs when both parties are satisfied with the outcome, and lose-lose is when neither party gets what they want. Nurse managers are challenged to build positive interdisciplinary work teams, and the process usually requires conflict management and resolution. One group strategy nurses have used to manage conflict is collective bargaining, which is aimed at preventing total control by employers over work conditions, skill mix, and compensation.

LEARNING TOOLS

Self-Assessment: Power

Power Inventory

Introduction: Power is an important aspect of our personal and professional lives. Understanding your own level of comfort with power will help you gain support and resources in your work environment.

Directions: 1. Write a brief response to the statement under each item. 2. Circle a number on the continuum that best corresponds with how you view yourself.

(1 = strongly agree, 2 = moderately agree, 3 = agree, 4 = somewhat agree, 5 = disagree)

1. I am sensitive to where power exists in organizations. 1 2 3 4 5

2. I feel that power can be used effectively without disadvantaging individuals. 1 2 3 4 5

3. I feel comfortable taking risks. 1 2 3 4 5

4. I try to obtain additional resources in my work setting. 1 2 3 4 5

5. I engage in activities to strengthen my power base. 1 2 3 4 5

6. I avoid activities that will decrease my power. 1 2 3 4 5

7. I feel I have a base of colleagues whom I can count on to support my ideas or projects. 1 2 3 4 5

8. I enjoy taking charge of situations or projects to accomplish goals. 1 2 3 4 5

9. I enjoy speaking in front of groups, meeting new people, and being the center of attention. 1 2 3 4 5

10. I enjoy competing for resources with others. 1 2 3 4 5

Scoring: Review the scoring of each of the 10 questions. Count the number of items that you ranked high (3, 4, or 5). Were the majority of your rankings high? Examine the items that you scored high. If you scored many items high you probably do not feel comfortable gaining and using power. Focus on one or two items where you would like to gain confidence in gaining power. Identify activities that you can engage in to empower yourself in personal and professional interactions.

Self-Assessment: Conflict

Introduction: Conflict management is an important skill for nurses to acquire in order to build teams, to work in complex client care situations, and to obtain scarce resources. By evaluating your conflict management style, you can gain insight into what strategies have been effective methods for resolving conflict. Huber's Perceived Conflict Scale measures the conflict among hospital nurses.

The Perceived Conflict Scale

Purpose: To become aware of job conflict levels. If you do not work in a health care organization, rate the following assessment from the perspective of a student working in the clinical agency.

Directions: Read each question, and circle the number that most accurately represents your feelings. Select option 3 if conflict exists, but you are unable to identify its strength. Each item has a 5-point Likert-type scale: 1 = strongly disagree, 2 = disagree, 3 = neutral, 4 = agree, and 5 = strongly agree.

	Strongly Disagree	Disagree	Neutral	Agree	Strongly Agree
1. Other nurses often disagree with each other about how work on this unit should be handled.	1	2	3	4	5
2. I usually agree with the way other nurses think things should be done on this unit.	1	2	3	4	5
3. My supervisor and I usually agree about what my job is and the requirements I must fulfill.	1	2	3	4	5
4. I usually agree with the decisions my head nurse and supervisor make.	1	2	3	4	5
5. Clients often demand that I do things I simply cannot do.	1	2	3	4	5
6. When I do something that satisfies one person or group, other people are frequently upset with what I have done.	1	2	3	4	5
7. The employees that I see who are from other areas of the hospital are often difficult to deal with.	1	2	3	4	5
8. The various departments that I deal with in the hospital are usually helpful and make it easy for me to do my job.	1	2	3	4	5
9. I frequently encounter problems when I transfer my clients to other units or departments.	1	2	3	4	5
10. Support services (dietary, maintenance, etc.) are readily available when I need them.	1	2	3	4	5
11. Many times, the things that support services are supposed to do are not adequately done, and I either have to argue with another unit or do someone else's job.	1	2	3	4	5
12. I am unable to provide adequate client care because of the time that I spend dealing with hospital rules and red tape.	1	2	3	4	5
13. I often cannot get equipment, supplies, or medications when I need them.	1	2	3	4	5
14. My clients often make requests or need care that I feel I should provide, but cannot because I lack the time or energy.	1	2	3	4	5
15. My obligations to my work frequently conflict with my obligations to family, friends, or myself (outside the job).	1	2	3	4	5
16. I often have too many things to do at one time.	1	2	3	4	5

Reverse Score Items: For items 2, 3, 4, 8, and 10 reverse the 1-5 Likert scale to score them. For example, if you scored 5, change it to 1; if you scored 1, change it to 5; if you scored 4, change it to 2; and if you scored 2, change it to 4.

Subscales: Name	Items

1. Intrapersonal Conflict 5, 14, 15, 16
   *Conflict that arises within the individual from two competing demands.
2. Interpersonal Conflict 1, 2, 3, 4
   *Conflict between two or more individuals arising from miscommunication or differences in values.
3. Intergroup/Support Conflict 10, 11, 12, 13
   *Conflict between two or more groups that are supportive in work or personal lives. Differences in competition for resources, power, or status may occur.
4. Intergroup/Other Departments 6, 7, 8, 9
   *Conflict between two or more groups for resources or services. The conflict may be competitive or disruptive and may center around resources or control.

***Scoring:** The higher the mean score, the greater the level of conflict.

CASE STUDY: POWER

Sandy, a staff nurse on a 66-bed medical-surgical unit in Sagers, Hawaii, decides to establish a strong power base for herself. She has read a book about power mechanisms and decides to experiment with them. Sandy arrives on the unit and notices that her assignment is heavy. She decides to address the charge nurse by stating the facts about the number of clients she has, and their acuity levels. She requests that the assignment be adjusted in light of the data presented. The charge nurse refuses Sandy's request and walks away. Sandy decides to approach the nurse manager and again presents all the facts. The nurse manager intervenes and modifies the assignment. Sandy meets Ruth Ann, a clinical nurse specialist, in the hall and praises her for the new client care delivery model she developed. Finally, Sandy begins care delivery and realizes she cannot handle the turning and positioning alone. She seeks assistance from Judy and says she will return the favor. Judy agrees to help.

Case Study Questions

1. What power mechanisms did Sandy use?
2. Is Sandy empowering herself by using these power mechanisms?
3. What else can Sandy do to garner power?

CASE STUDY: CONFLICT

Jennifer is a nurse manager on a neuroscience unit in Chicago, Illinois. She has been trying to get funding for renovating the neuroscience unit. Jonathan is a nurse manager on the orthopedic unit in the same hospital. The vice president of nursing has announced that there is enough money to renovate only one unit in the hospital, and that she would like proposals from both Jennifer and Jonathan because their units are those in the most need for repair. Jennifer calls Jonathan after the meeting and asks if they could meet and discuss the renovation issue. Jonathan eagerly accepts the invitation since he has wanted to work with Jennifer to resolve this conflict of interest.

Jennifer and Jonathan meet with a detailed work plan of desired renovations for each of their units. They both have costs for the projects. Jennifer and Jonathan both agree that they do not want to compete for the renovation because morale will suffer greatly on the unit that loses. The two units adjoin, and they freely share staff back and forth as the census demands. Jennifer and Jonathan brainstorm and come up with several options, such as rebidding the work based on two units that are adjacent (perhaps they could get a discount); renovating the units in phases, part one this year and part two the next; or perhaps if this was not possible, renovating one unit this year and purchasing new equipment for the other unit and then reversing the process. Jennifer and Jonathan make a joint appointment to speak with the vice president of nursing.

Case Study Questions

1. What type of conflict outcome were Jennifer and Jonathan attempting to elicit?
2. What types of conflict strategies were Jennifer and Jonathan using?
3. What type of framework for conflict strategy were Jennifer and Jonathan using to get their desired outcome?

LEARNING RESOURCES

Discussion Questions

1. What are the five power bases described by French and Raven?
2. What is the difference between personal power-oriented individuals and institutionalized power-oriented individuals?
3. How can a nurse manager empower the staff? What effect does empowerment have on care delivery?
4. What are effective strategies for staff nurses to use to empower themselves and their colleagues?
5. What are the differences between fight, negotiation, and collaboration? Identify a situation in which each might be appropriate.
6. Describe and discuss the three conflict resolution outcomes in terms of teambuilding and long-term positive relationships among individuals competing for resources.

7. Discuss the use of conflict resolution strategies, and identify the outcome possible when using each of the strategies.
8. How can nurses as a group work together to have significant impact on legislative issues affecting nursing practice?
9. Is collective bargaining useful in nursing? What is the purpose of collective bargaining and how can it be useful to nurses? How can it inhibit the nursing profession's growth?
10. What are sources of conflict in nursing and what can nurses do to resolve this conflict and promote growth?

Study Questions

Matching: Write the correct letter of the correct response in front of each term.

_____ 1. Power
_____ 2. Empowerment
_____ 3. Reward power
_____ 4. Coercive power
_____ 5. Expert power
_____ 6. Referent power
_____ 7. Legitimate power
_____ 8. Ingratiation
_____ 9. Upward appeal
_____ 10. Coalitions

A. Power based on charisma and interpersonal appeal
B. The authority to act based on position
C. Providing the opportunity for others to take responsibility and accountability for their work
D. Influencing an individual or group in order to gain a scarce resource
E. Lavishing praise on another in order to gain favor
F. Formation of a group for the purpose of a single voice in order to affect change
G. Taking concern to a higher authority
H. The use of threats, discipline, or negative consequences
I. Individuals who possess special skills or talents
J. Providing a pay raise, promotion, or advancement

True or False: Circle the correct answer.

T F 1. Conflict arises because job descriptions are clear, policies and procedures are written, and growth is fostered in an organization.

T F 2. Organizational conflict arises from the competition for scarce resources.

T F 3. In order to build effective interdisciplinary teams, conflict must be present, and managers must not interfere with conflict resolution.

T F 4. Role ambiguity is the expectation that nurses take on duties from other disciplines.

T F 5. People are most comfortable around people who are like them.

T F 6. A defensive framework for conflict resolution includes winning some resources and losing others.

T F 7. Using the conflict strategy of withdrawing provides the participant with the time to calm down or avoid confrontation.

T F 8. In a win-lose situation, both parties end up losing because nobody is one hundred percent satisfied.

T F 9. Collective bargaining is used by nurses to prevent management from making all of the decisions without input from the nurses about compensation and workload.

T F 10. Role stress occurs when the nurse's responsibilities expand faster than the formal job description.

SUPPLEMENTAL READINGS

Drory, A. & Ritov, I. (1997). Effects of work experience and opponent's power on conflict management styles. *International Journal of Conflict Management, 8(2)*, 148-161.

Gilbert, T. (1998). Toward a politics of trust. *Journal of Advanced Nursing, 27(5)*, 1010-1016.

King, C. & Koliner, A. (1999). Understanding the impact of power in organizations. *Seminars for Nurse Managers, 7(1)*, 39-46.

Pondy, L. (1967). Organizational conflict: Concepts and models. *Administrative Science Quarterly, 12*, 296-320.

Varman, R. & Bhatnagar, D. (1999). Power and politics in grievance resolution. *Human Relations, 52(3)*, 349-382.

ANSWERS TO TEXT STUDY QUESTIONS

Chapter 10—Power and Conflict (p. 199)

1. **Pick a day in the past couple of weeks that you think of as average. Who were the people who had the most influence over you? Why were they influential?**

   You may have identified co-workers, family members, and fellow students as people who have influenced your life. What strategies did they enlist to exert their influence? Did they use assertiveness, ingratiation, rationality, sanctions, exchange, upward appeal, blocking, or coalitions? Were they influential because you felt guilty, motivated, encouraged, or defeated?

2. **Do you view power as positive or negative? Give examples.**

   One's perception of power is influenced by one's position, privilege, knowledge, and experience. While many nurses view power as unconstructive or bad, power is not inherently negative. Positive power exerts influence on behalf of others while negative power exerts influence over others. What have your experiences been? How do you react to those exerting power over you?

3. **Identify the kinds of power you use and the kinds of power others use on you.**

   To help you address this issue, consider the following questions: What is your belief regarding your personal power? Do you believe that you can influence events through personal effort? How about professional power? Do you get rewards from doing a job, acquiring expertise, being liked, and having charisma? Do you have the power to use your professional expertise and competence to make changes, do something good for clients, advance the profession, or make a contribution? What are the strengths of power used by those you respect?

4. **What types of power are you most comfortable with? Which would you consider trying?**

   There are many sources of power. Are you more comfortable with reward power, coercive power, expert power, referent power, legitimate power, connection power, and group decision-making power? In what situation might you use each? Which sources of power are you least comfortable exercising? Which are you the most comfortable exercising? Why do you think you feel that way?

5. **Think about yourself as acting with strength and power and feeling the most satisfied about it. What kinds of things would you be doing?**

   It is important to analyze what gives you a sense of power. Nurses may be inclined to avoid an acknowledgment or analysis of power. However, to lead and manage, nurses need to acquire, possess, and use power effectively. Nurses may use power to improve client outcomes, to advance the nursing profession, and to improve the organizational climate.

6. **What happens in situations in which you feel powerless?**

   Individuals may react differently when facing powerless situations. A loss of control may precipitate emotions such as fear, anxiety, and anger. Behaviors such as withdrawal and aggression may also be exhibited. How do you react when you feel powerless? Do you withdraw, fight, negotiate, or collaborate? Do you develop behaviors that are counterproductive to the organization? How do you regain a sense of power?

7. **Does a lack of power affect the way that you feel about situations?**

   A lack of power may negatively affect the way one feels about a given situation. Powerless situations may result in passive participation, work dissatisfaction, and diminished productivity. Prolonged feelings of powerlessness may lead to demoralization and depression. How do you perceive your attitude in powerless situations? How could you modify your outlook to regain a sense of power?

8. **When you are trying to control a situation, what makes you feel comfortable or uncomfortable?**

   Attempting to control a situation may cause an individual to use power to control others, rather than to empower others to improve the situation. How a person responds to a power conflict is related to their personality, experience, position, perspective, and the problem. Which approach do you take when faced with power conflicts?

9. **How can power principles be structured to advance nursing's professional goals?**

   Nurses can use power principles to establish a foundation that will enlist support to advance the image, power, and prestige of nursing. Each nurse has the power to project enthusiasm, self-confidence, and self-esteem. Professional introductions and the display of academic credentials are two ways that nurses can reinforce their image. Power is also derived from the art and science of nursing practice. Nurses can use expertise, information, and nursing research data to render cost-effective client care.

10. What is the difference, if any, between power and manipulation?

Similarities exist between the concepts of power and manipulation. One view of power is the ability to get others to do what you want done. Manipulation is commonly viewed as controlling others by artful, unfair, or insidious means.

11. How is organizational power used?

Organizational power is often seen as control over valuable resources. Sources of power in organizations are structural positions, personal characteristics, expertise, and opportunity. Organizational power implies the ability to mobilize support, information, and resources in order to meet organizational goals. Power is also used as a mechanism to resolve conflict. Employees with access to power and opportunity feel empowered to contribute to the organization, participate more actively, and exhibit higher morale.

12. What was the most recent conflict you experienced?

Consider the type of conflict you experienced. Was it intrapersonal, interpersonal, or intergroup? What were the antecedent conditions that led you to perceive and feel conflict? What was your manifest behavior? What was the conflict aftermath? Did you perceive the conflict to be positive or negative?

13. What types of conflict are common in nursing students?

Nursing students may experience intrapersonal, interpersonal, or intergroup conflicts. Intrapersonal conflict may result as nursing students try to juggle multiple and competing roles, such as parent, spouse, student, and friend. An interpersonal conflict may erupt between a student and faculty member over a paper or project due date. An intergroup conflict may occur among a group of nursing students working on a project if it is perceived that the workload is not equally divided.

14. What sources of conflict are most common in nursing practice?

Nurses may experience conflict because of the need to work collaboratively with individuals with different values, beliefs, and perspectives. Conflicts may arise from differences in communication styles, goals, expectations, resources, and roles. Power distribution for nurses employed in a hierarchical system may lead to conflicts as they attempt to meet the needs of their clients and advocate for scarce resources to provide the care.

15. What is your usual way of handling conflict?

Consider which mode you find yourself in when a conflict surfaces. Are you in the defensive mode? Do you tend to compromise? Do you enlist creative problem solving techniques? Conflict resolution techniques include avoiding, withholding or withdrawing, smoothing over or reassuring, accommodating, forcing, competing, compromising, confronting, collaborating, bargaining and negotiating, and problem solving. Which are your preferred techniques? What others might you try?

16. What is the usual way nurses handle conflict?

Depending on working relationships, bureaucratic hierarchy, and differences in power, nurses may use a variety of techniques to handle conflict. These techniques include avoidance, accommodation, compromise, competition, collaboration, and problem solving. The degree of assertiveness and cooperativeness may vary with the given situation, the technique selected, and the comfort level of the nurse(s).

17. Does the way your immediate superior handles conflict help or hinder you?

Think about the conflict resolution outcomes achieved by your immediate supervisor. Are they win-lose, lose-lose, or win-win? How is the conflict framed? Is conflict viewed constructively from the perspective of increasing group cohesion and morale, promoting creativity, producing change and growth, improving work relationships, promoting effective problem solving, and motivating group members? Or is conflict viewed as a destructive force that interferes with stability and harmony?

18. Is there one best way to handle the conflicts most common to nursing practice?

A variety of strategies can be employed to handle conflicts in nursing. It is important to conduct an assessment of the conflict situation in order to identify the parameters of the conflict, areas of agreement and disagreement, and person's perspective and goals. The factors that limit the possibilities of managing the conflict constructively must be communicated, explicated, and resolved.

Communication, Persuasion, and Negotiation

STUDY FOCUS

Communication is an essential element in organizing, coordinating, and directing the care of clients. Nurse managers are challenged to create clear communication pathways to facilitate task accomplishment in organizations. *Communication* is the ability to transmit information to another clearly. *Organizational communication* is the ability of an agency to transmit information to and from its members expediently and expeditiously. *Verbal communication* is verbal or written information, and nonverbal communication is transmitted through behaviors. The four distinctions in communication are those between the formal/informal, vertical/horizontal, personal/impersonal, and instrumental/expressive types. *Formal communication* is the official information sent by designated officials in an agency, and informal is information passed via the grapevine. *Vertical communication* is boss to employee, and *horizontal* is peer to peer. *Personal communication* is when mutual influence occurs, and impersonal is one-sided communication. *Instrumental communication* is transmitting data essential to complete work, and expressive is data that is tangential to the work that is done.

Communication is both an art and a skill in which a sender and a receiver engage in the transmission of ideas or information. The steps in communication whereby information is exchanged include the following: First, there is message formulation where the sender formulates the ideas; second, the message is encoded and the sender formulates the idea into verbal or nonverbal components; third, the message is transmitted and the sender imparts the message; fourth, the receiver acquires the transmission and the message is received by the selected method; and finally, the process is completed when the message is decoded and the receiver interprets the data.

In communication, there is always the potential for barriers due to the perception and filtration of information by both the sender and receiver. People have their own unique world view, which colors or changes the message to fit their model of the world. Therefore, it is extremely important to keep messages clear, simple, and relevant to the receiver.

Group communication is even more complex than individual communication because of the number of individuals involved. Five common communication networks are used: the wheel, the chain, the Y, the all-channel, and the circle. In centralized organizations, the wheel, the Y, and the chain are used. In democratic organizations the circle and the all-channel networks are used most often.

There are five basic internal organizational communication systems that include downward, upward, horizontal, grapevine, and network communications. Formal communication channels include downward, upward, and horizontal modes. *Informal communication* channels include the grapevine and network. *Networks* include a group of people who come together to socialize or work on a team. Communication styles that facilitate communication include affirming, listening, nonaggressive, confident, and indirect approaches. Effective aspects of business communication include brief, simple, and straightforward communications that are receiver-centered (Katz & Green, 1997).

Communication effectiveness is influenced by the message, the way it is delivered, and the method used to communicate. People tend to respond more positively when they are contacted individually. Discrimination or exclusion raises sensitivities and distracts from the message. It is important to determine if the receiver understands the message. Feedback is an important managerial tool and enhances subordinates' performance. Clear, immediate, honest input is required for effective outcomes.

Because they work in complex, technologically advanced environments with people who are not well, nurses have typically been targets of criticism from clients, physicians, and other health care workers. Strategies for dealing with critical individuals include agreeing with the criticism, seeking further information, and guiding the criticism toward problem solving. At times, managers must use constructive criticism in order to improve subordinates' performance. In these cases, blame should not be the focus; instead the focus should be on analysis of the problems and a formulation of goals to be achieved in order to solve them. Constructive feedback should be given in an appropriate environment and time. Specific behavioral statements should be used to describe the problem behavior.

Nurses must also remember that image is important in communicating professionalism to the public. Dress and appearance significantly affect the public's perception of the nurse's image. Nurses can use language to clearly articulate their values and the nature of their work with clients.

Conflict is inevitable. Nurses must learn effective strategies to resolve conflict and enhance collaborative efforts among interdisciplinary team members. Two powerful tools that may resolve conflicts are persuasion and negotiation. Individuals use persuasion to get what they want when they believe coercion is unethical. Bargaining and negotiation are also useful in resolving a conflict.

Persuasion is the ability to influence others to change their behavior based on argument or reasoning. An individual skillful at persuasion will leave the listener with some perception of choice. Persuaders have a variety of motives for their approach, with the most typical being self-preservation, money, romance, or recognition. Effective communication is essential when attempting to persuade others. In the course of persuasion, timing, strategy, and credibility are important in the attempt to lower listeners' defenses, as well as in complimenting, and supporting them. Commitment, imagination, and trust are three elements crucial to successful persuasion.

The five reasons for exerting influence are to obtain assistance, to get others to do their job, to obtain personal benefits, to initiate change, and to improve job performance. Assertiveness, ingratiation, rationality, sanctions, exchange, upward appeal, blocking, and coalitions are all influence tactics. In effective persuasion, two tactics are frequently used. They include the emphasizing certain points and downplaying other points. Important persuasive techniques are using repetition, creating miscommunication, and providing rational explanations, while avoiding threats and fear tactics.

Negotiation is the give-and-take exchange among individuals who want to resolve conflict in a way acceptable to all parties involved. *Bargaining* is closely related to negotiation and is the exchange of favors among individuals. *Collective bargaining* is a type of negotiation governed by specific laws and rules. Individuals engage in negotiation to prevent win-lose situations. In order to classify an interaction as a negotiation, the following three criteria must be present: the issue must be negotiable; the negotiators must be willing to give and take; and the individuals must trust each other and the process. Four elements in the negotiation process are the goals, values, mutual victory, and incomplete information.

There are ten steps in the negotiation process. The first step is preparing for the negotiation. The second step is communicating a general overview of what is to be accomplished in the negotiation. Third, the reasons why each party feels the negotiation is necessary should be reviewed. Fourth, the parties should redefine and clarify the issue(s). Fifth, the parties should agree on the agenda and select when in the course of meeting the issues will be addressed. In the sixth step, discussion should be encouraged and facilitated throughout the negotiation process. During discussions, the seventh step, an exploration of the compromise positions for both parties should be examined. Eighth, during the settlement stage, each party should agree in principle to the solution or possible solutions for the issue. Ninth, a thorough review and summarizing of the agreement should take place. Finally, a process should be established and implemented to monitor the parties' compliance and progress with the final agreement.

Formal negotiations have a specialized language that individuals use to convey the activities that occur throughout the process. Terms such as issues, deadlock or stalemate, impasse, concessions, power, flinch, deadline, and nibble are used. Issues refer to negotiable items or to those conflicts which need to be resolved. An *impasse* is a point in time when issues cannot be resolved. Impasses lead to deadlocks or stalemates in which individuals are unable to reach agreement. *Concessions* refer to favors given or positions changed in order to continue negotiations or to provide a satisfactory settlement to all parties. They are those items that are of little or no value to you, but important to others and can be used strategically to influence the negotiation process. *Power* is the ability to influence others. A *flinch* is to express displeasure with the initial proposal in order to begin the negotiation process. A *deadline* is an end date on a schedule used to keep both parties on target and progressing in the negotiation process. A *nibble* is a small concession after the agreement has been settled.

Preparation for negotiations is essential for success. The ability to determine the parameters for negotiation helps control the issues and areas of discussion. Dressing professionally and being aware of both verbal and nonverbal messages are important in resolving issues and tipping off the opposing party. Good listening skills and a positive communication tone are essential for effective negotiation. Maintaining a flexible position is also important in a successful negotiation.

Nurses have unionized for a variety of reasons. Some of the more recent issues sparking unionization efforts include layoffs, the reduction of hours, elimination of incentives, the cessation of pay increases, and the denial of benefits. The use of UAPs in place of RNs and the increasing number of employees a clinical nurse must supervise have sparked concerns about unsafe client care and inadequate staffing levels. To verbalize the concerns of nurses to management, nurses have occasionally turned to unionization as a method of strengthening their voice and demanding accountability for unilateral administrative decisions influencing client care.

LEARNING TOOLS

Group Activity: Exploring Verbal and Nonverbal Communication

Purpose: To identify the impact of verbal and nonverbal communication when interacting with others. In light of the fact that approximately 55% of a speaker's message is the result of facial and body language (the majority is facial); 38% the vocal quality; and only 7% the actual words used, this activity is designed to help you assess your communication style with others.

Directions: Divide yourselves into groups of three. One person will be sending a message; one person will be receiving the message; and one person will observe the interaction and then provide feedback. First, have one person describe the most important thing that has happened to him or her within the past year. Three minutes should be allowed for the interaction. Then reverse the procedure until everyone has had an opportunity to observe, send, and receive a message. Observers should jot down comments about verbal and nonverbal communication. The following observer checklist may be used. Second, have each person describe the worst thing that has happened to him or her in the last year. Again, use the observer checklist to record comments.

Afterward, everyone should share his or her observer comments with the group. Talk with each other about the impact verbal and nonverbal communication have on the content of the message. Receivers should discuss the verbal or nonverbal activity that they focused on the most. Discuss how mannerisms or nonverbal behaviors can distract or support a message.

Observer Checklist

For each of the categories, prompts are provided. Write down the major and minor verbal and nonverbal characteristics that you noted for both the sender and receiver.

Facial Expression

1. Note the eyes and mouth for expressiveness. Is the sender relating happiness? sadness?
2. How is the receiver responding?

Sender Receiver

Body Language

1. Note the arms, hands, legs, shoulders, and hips. How is the sender illustrating his or her message?
2. How is the receiver acknowledging the message?
3. Is the sender's message supportive, disinterested, or boring?
4. What impact is the sender's message having on the receiver? Is the sender changing the content of the message based on the receiver's feedback?

Sender Receiver

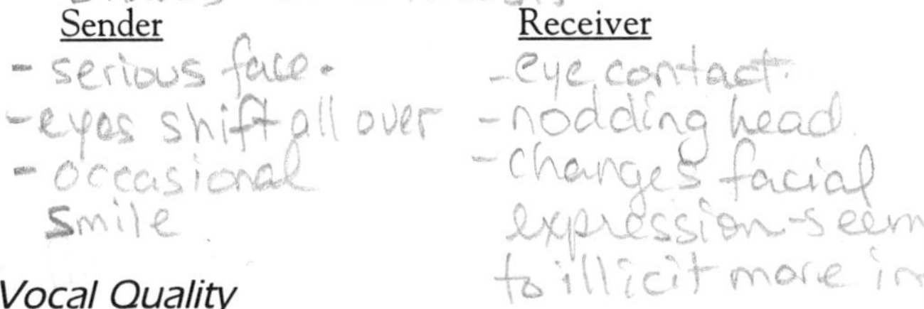

Vocal Quality

1. Is the tone, pitch, and volume consistent with the message?
2. Is the sender's message spoken in a monotone? Is there variation in tone to make an impact on the receiver?
3. Is the sender forceful? weak? bored? interested? animated? eager?
4. Does the sender use a strong, soft, reflective, or humorous presentation?

Sender Receiver

Articulated Words

1. What actual verbal message was sent?
2. What words were used to send the message?
3. Were metaphors used? Were red flags or emotionally charged words used?

Sender Receiver

Role Play #1

Using Persuasion to Influence Others

Character One = Jennifer is the vice president of nursing at a large teaching hospital in Topeka, Kansas. She has decided to organize a team to work on critical pathways and to then implement them in the hospital in an effort to provide cost-effective, high-quality care to clients.

Character Two = Jason is the chief executive officer (CEO) of the hospital. He is very concerned about rising costs and is tightening up on resources. He plans to hold the line and not distribute money for new projects that cannot guarantee a payoff.

Character Three = Joe is the vice president of building and maintenance. He is over budget on a new building project and needs additional money to finish the new building. He plans to speak to Jason to secure the needed funds.

Character Four = Mary Ann is the chief financial officer (CFO). She has crunched some figures and is prepared to speak to Jason about the bottom line. She has designed a forecasted projection of the next six months' revenue and expenses, and she is prepared to make recommendations about cost cutting to ensure organizational viability.

• • • • •

Jennifer has entered Jason's office prepared to share with him a new project (critical pathways) that would improve quality and decrease costs. She knows that there will be an initial outlay of money, but is sure that there will be a major payoff for the organization. As she turns the corner toward Jason's office, she sees Mary Ann and Joe talking. Jason opens his door and sees his executive team waiting to speak to him.

Role-Play Questions

1. What should Jennifer do? Should she take the lead and jump right in with her new idea? If so, what should she say? How should she introduce the topic?
2. What persuasive techniques should Jennifer use to elicit support for her project?
3. How could she persuade others to support her project and yet support them with their plans?

CASE STUDY: MANAGING FEEDBACK

Martha is the nurse manager of an operating room in Lake Worth, Florida. Jill is a registered nurse who has worked in the operating room for three years. Lately, Jill has been having problems completing the documentation that she is required to do, has been taking long breaks, and is refusing to scrub for several physicians. Martha is informed that staffing is short and that they will need her to cover cases just to get through the day. Martha enjoys scrubbing and is very willing to help out to facilitate a smooth progression of clients through the operating room. After Martha has finished her second case, the charge nurse informs her that they are one case behind. Martha asks if there was an emergency or a late case. The charge nurse says no, but that Jill took a 45-minute break and refused to scrub for a physician. Martha walks into the conference room where Jill is reading a book. Martha angrily reprimands Jill in front of two staff members and tells Jill to either scrub for the physician or go home.

Case Study Questions

1. Did Martha respond in an appropriate fashion?
2. What other strategies could Martha have used to manage this situation?
3. What are characteristics of constructive feedback?

CASE STUDY: COMMUNICATION—PERSUASION AND NEGOTIATION

Jennifer is a nurse manager of an ambulatory care clinic in a large teaching hospital. The ambulatory care clinic is very successful and is a good revenue source for the hospital. Recently, the physicians and nurse practitioners in the ambulatory care clinic negotiated a contract with a large employer in the community to provide primary care for all of their employees. The contract was negotiated at a discounted rate. The physicians and nurse practitioners have held a team conference to look at expenses, workload, and equipment usage. They have asked Jennifer to figure out a way to use the RNs more effectively, and if necessary, to hire medical assistants. Jennifer knows that the nurses will resist. She also knows that the RNs could be utilized more effectively in client teaching activities, immunizations, and triage.

Case Study Questions

1. What should Jennifer do? Should she be autocratic and demand that the RNs comply? Should she use persuasion to get them to do what she wants? Should she negotiate with them?
2. If Jennifer chooses to use persuasion, should she listen to their concerns?
3. If Jennifer chooses to use negotiation and a settlement is agreed upon, who is responsible for evaluating and monitoring progress?

LEARNING RESOURCES

Discussion Questions

1. What is essential for effective communication to occur?

2. What types of communication networks are there? What types of communication networks are used in decentralized and centralized organizations?
3. What are the steps in information exchange?
4. Why are nurses targeted for criticism? What strategies can nurses use to handle criticism?
5. What are the current issues in health care organizations today that nurses might choose to unionize in order to have a strong collective voice?
6. Describe the process of negotiation that nurses could use to address pressing issues in client care with administrative personnel.
7. Are persuasion, negotiation, and bargaining useful in both personal and professional interactions? If so, provide an example of each for both a personal and professional situation.
8. What is the difference between coercion and persuasion? Should both be used? If so, why? If not, why not?

Study Questions

True or False: Circle the correct answer.

T F 1. Verbal communication includes both affective and expressive behaviors.

T F 2. Positive communication techniques include agreeing uncritically and reassuringly.

T F 3. Individual communication is more complex than group communication because it is so intensive.

T F 4. Horizontally decentralized organizations are more efficient than centralized organizations.

T F 5. Feedback should be used carefully and only when absolutely necessary since it inhibits effective communication.

T F 6. To respond effectively to communication, place blame on others.

T F 7. The major part of any communication is the words we say to others.

T F 8. Effective communication is clear, direct, and straightforward.

T F 9. Metaphors and political language can be used by nurse leaders to influence governmental officials.

T F 10. Nurses are often targets of verbal abuse.

Matching: Write the letter of the correct response in front of each term.

_____ 1. Negotiation
_____ 2. Bargaining
_____ 3. Persuasion
_____ 4. Collective bargaining
_____ 5. Flinch
_____ 6. Nibble
_____ 7. Concessions
_____ 8. Deadline
_____ 9. Impasse
_____ 10. Issues

A. A small extra item that is obtained after the settlement
B. Items of little value to one party
C. A point in time when issues cannot be resolved to mutual satisfaction
D. Items to be resolved
E. Activities governed by law and rules
F. Influencing another to modify behaviors
G. Time frames for negotiations
H. To draw back at an initial proposal
I. Give-and-take exchange aimed at resolving conflicts
J. The exchange of favors

REFERENCE

Katz, J.M. & Green, E. (1997). *Managing quality: A guide to system-wide performance management in health care* (2nd Ed.). St. Louis: Mosby.

SUPPLEMENTAL READINGS

Johnson, J. (1998). Managers' forum. Financial negotiation. *Journal of Emergency Nursing, 24(4)*, 348-349.

Mariono, T.Y. & Kahnoski, B. (1998). Communication action for casemanagers: Techniques to manage conflict. *Nursing Case Management, 3(1)*, 36-45.

Milligan, R.A., Gilroy, J., Katz, K.S., Rodan, M.F. & Subramanian, K.N. (1999). Developing a shared language: Interdisciplinary communication among diverse health care professionals. *Holistic Nursing Practice 13(2)*, 47-53.

O'Mara, K. (1999). Communication and conflict resolution in emergency medicine. *Emergency Medicine Clinics of North America, 17(2)*, 451-459.

Wyatt, D. (1999). Negotiation strategies for men and women. *Nursing Management, 30(1)*, 22-26.

ANSWERS TO TEXT STUDY QUESTIONS

Chapter 11—Communication, Persuasion, and Negotiation (pp. 226–227)

1. **What are the essential components of the communication process?**

The communication process consists of verbal and nonverbal communication. Verbal communication is both written and spoken. Nonverbal communication is unspoken and is composed of affective or expressive behaviors. There are four distinctions of communication: formal and informal, vertical and horizontal, personal and impersonal, and instrumental and expressive.

2. **What are the barriers to effective communication in organizations?**

Barriers to effective communication in organizations include political and interpersonal subtleties and the complexity of communicating with multiple people. Organizations use various systems for communication such as hierarchical or democratic networks. Barriers in the hierarchical network may be associated with decreased opportunity for individuals to interact with their peers or people on other levels in the hierarchy. Barriers in the democratic network may be associated with communication inaccuracy and the development of subhierarchies.

3. **What problems of communication occur frequently in nursing?**

Both verbal and nonverbal communication problems occur in nursing. These problems frequently center on issues of competency, responsibility, and professionalism and may be related to being on the front lines, being the focus for displaced criticism, working with people who have health problems, and working in high-stress environments. Nonverbal communication problems exist when the media portrays an unprofessional image of nursing.

4. **Are employer-employee communication problems more common than peer-to-peer difficulties?**

It is equally common to experience communication problems in employer-employee and peer-to-peer relationships. Problems associated with employer-employee communications may be the result of intimidation, mistrust, insufficient feedback, or the inability to articulate needs. Similarly, peer-to-peer miscommunications may be the result of lack of trust or a difficulty with needs expression, but may also encompass an inability to give and receive constructive criticism and turf issues.

5. **What solutions tend to help communication effectiveness?**

Planning the message structure, delivery style, mode of communication, and method for feedback can enhance communication effectiveness. Planning the message involves structuring it so that it will be positively received and will engender the desired response. The selection of delivery style includes careful selection of words to maximize the desired impact. The mode of communication involves decisions about the timing and the optimal vehicle for transmission. The method for feedback includes a plan for determining if the delivered message was understood. Solutions for responding effectively to criticism include soliciting additional input, clarifying the issues, agreeing with the critic, and using listening skills to enhance understanding.

6. **What is the relationship of communication skill to leadership effectiveness?**

Communication skill is a key element of leadership effectiveness. It is a critical and important tool for engaging, motivating, and empowering people to accomplish organizational goals. The skill of communication is essential in sharing the vision, in shaping the organizational culture, and in implementing change.

7. **What is the leader's role in helping others improve written and oral communication?**

The leader plays an important role in mentoring others to improve their communication skills. This can be accomplished through a variety of methods, such as role modeling, soliciting and providing constructive criticism, and role-playing. It is critical for the leader to model a communication style that is clear, direct, honest, respectful, empathetic, and timely.

8. **How important is written communication skill in influencing an individual's image?**

Written communication skill is an important professional element that impacts an individual's image. Organizations commonly transmit information in the form of fliers, memos, letters, faxes, e-mail, and newsletters. Skill is required to structure a clear and concise written message that will be positively received. Unclear written messages may present ambiguous information that increases the likelihood for misunderstanding.

9. How do you personally communicate, both verbally and nonverbally?

One's personal communication style may incorporate verbal and nonverbal components. Individuals communicate to others through their appearance, body language, diction, language, mannerism, tone, volume, and word selection. It is important to be aware of your communication strengths and weaknesses and how others receive your intended message.

10. How might you choose some other message or some other channel to increase your personal effectiveness?

Consider your message structure. Are you consciously thinking about whether it will be positively received and if it will elicit the desired response? Are your words clear and free from red flags, inflammatory language, and jargon? Are you aware of the nonverbal communications that you portray? Before selecting a communication channel, it is important to think about the advantages and disadvantages associated with written and spoken communication.

11. Do nurses, from the staff nurse to the chief nurse executive, present an image of nursing that you agree or disagree with?

Think about the image of nursing that you value. Is there consensus or discord among others regarding the image? Do your peers and colleagues agree with the image? How about health care consumers? Do you hold a different image of nursing for the staff nurse and the chief nurse executive? Should you?

12. What does the ideal nurses' uniform look like? Analyze your response.

The ideal nurses' uniform is one that conveys a professional appearance and allows the nurse to carry out her or his duties and responsibilities. While there is consensus that a nurse's uniform should be comfortable and identifiable, disagreement continues over the color and style of the garment. Research has shown that health care consumers prefer white uniforms, in contrast to nurses, who prefer scrubs outfits. How would you blend the two perspectives to meet the needs of both groups? Are they mutually exclusive? Are the preferences of one group more important than the other?

13. Why do nurses need to look professional?

Physical appearance and choice of clothing are forms of nonverbal communication that others use to formulate judgments. A professional appearance enhances the image of nursing, influencing the amount of trust, confidence, and prestige that consumers, colleagues, and corporations afford them.

14. What persuades individuals to become a nurse?

A variety of factors may influence an individual's decision to become a nurse. For example, some may be drawn to nursing for altruistic reasons or for the excitement of working in a fast-paced health care environment. Still others are drawn to nursing for job security, professional advancement and challenge, and research opportunities.

15. What feelings are associated with an interview for a nursing position?

An interview for a nursing position is a process in which applicants seeking employment attempt to persuade the interviewer that they are the best candidates for the position. Applicants may experience feelings of anxiousness, nervousness, excitement, or apprehension during the interview process.

16. What was the last issue you negotiated?

Analyze your negotiation process. What was the central issue in the negotiation? What were your objectives or goals? What were the goals of the other person? How did the goals vary with respect to urgency and priority as the negotiation efforts continued? Was it a win-win, win-lose, or lose-lose result? What information was withheld in order to maintain a sense of negotiating power?

17. What behaviors contribute to cooperative and productive negotiation?

Cooperative and productive negotiation can only occur if the issue is negotiable, the negotiators are interested in compromising, and if there is mutual trust and cooperation. In a supportive environment, negotiation is problem-focused and sincere. Successful negotiation depends on the participants being well prepared, their use of effective communication skills, a willingness to take calculated risks, and to work toward a mutually supported solution.

18. What words or actions indicate competitive negotiation?

A competitive negotiation process may have a defense milieu in which there are feelings of superiority and domination. Indications of competitive negotiation include ineffective communication, stressful reactions, personal agendas, and unrevealed information. Information may be altered, filtered, given selectively, or withheld as a power gaining strategy. Questions may be framed to lead the other party to the competitor's point of view rather than to genuinely seek understanding.

19. What approaches or strategies of negotiation are most effective for nursing?

While there are numerous negotiation strategies available for use by nurses, the most effective are those that are deliberately planned and actualized. Laser (1981) identified four significant strategies for negotiation: the flinch, the deadline, the nibble, and the concession. The flinch strategy involves wincing at the initial proposition by the other party in an effort to open the negotiation dialogue. The deadline strategy produces results, is advisable in every negotiation, and must be negotiated among interested parties. The nibble strategy is a small, extra settlement that is reached after a larger decision has been attained. The concession strategy involves giving the other party concessions that are valuable to them, but of little or no value to you. Concessions should be identified, used strategically, and recorded. Other recommended strategies for successful negotiation include separating the people from the problem; focusing on interests, not positions; inventing options for mutual agreement; and using objective criteria. An awareness of available strategies enhances the negotiator's ability to choose alternative approaches, augment effectiveness, and achieve desirable outcomes.

20. What factors are facilitators or barriers to collaboration among professionals?

Facilitators to collaboration among professionals include willingness to compromise, cooperate, and a willingness to work toward a solution that everyone can support. Client-centered goals can be achieved through mutual trust, respect, and acknowledgment of each discipline's contribution. Barriers to collaboration include turf protection, power issues, arrogance, ineffective communication, and defensiveness.

21. Does collective bargaining increase professionalism in nursing?

Some believe that collective bargaining increases professionalism in nursing by ensuring that nursing has a voice in decisions related to client care, working conditions, wages, benefits, and professional practice. Collective bargaining exists to limit employers' ability to take unilateral action. Others believe that collective bargaining limits professionalism by creating a defensive environment between nurses and employers.

22. What organizational factors are associated with unionization?

Organizational factors associated with unionization include unilateral decisions made by employers to reduce costs by downsizing, merging, restructuring, and reengineering the workforce. Threats to long-term job security and benefits, reduction in income, increased workload, and concerns over quality care have created an increase in unionization activities.

23. Is positional power eroding in nursing? With what forms of negotiation can nurses replace positional power?

Positional power, or legitimate power, relates to the role or position held by nurses in organizations. When organizations make unilateral decisions about issues impacting professional practice without the input of nurses, the nurses' professional power is diminished. Nurses may need to strengthen their expert and referent power to ensure that client advocacy occurs. Nurses may seek and use power to influence professional practice, ethical issues, and national health care policies. Nurses can use negotiation to determine how nursing care is practiced and delivered in organizations by establishing a collaborative environment where the goals of all parties are respected and valued.

Delegation

STUDY FOCUS

The complexity and cost-constrained nature of the health care delivery system necessitates a multidisciplinary, multilevel approach to the provision of client care. Nurses must learn to delegate effectively to coordinate multidisciplinary teams and to manage especially complex client cases. *Delegation* is the ability to accomplish tasks through other people while maintaining accountability. A *delegator* is an individual who assigns or delegates the task to another. A *delegate* is an individual who accepts the delegated task. To effectively delegate, the delegator must supervise the work by providing direction for task accomplishment, periodically checking on the progress, and then evaluating the outcome.

Delegation is not dumping unpleasant work on others, being bossy, or abdicating responsibility and accountability. Managers should not delegate personal accountability, the disciplining of employees, or the recognition and praise of good work to others. Delegation is used to improve others' skills, assign new tasks, build teams, and complete tasks that you do not have time to do. As a nurse, you will delegate both nursing activities, the tasks essential to provide client care, and non-nursing activities, the tasks necessary to support client care. The six basic principles of delegation are to know yourself and team members; assess the strengths, weaknesses, job description, and situation of yourself and your team members; know your state practice act; assess your job requirements; communicate clearly; and evaluate the outcome. The National Council of State Boards of Nursing (NCSBN) has developed tools and a decision-making process for delegation. The tool assists with assessing critical elements in delegation decisions. The critical elements include level of client, level of UAP competence, level of licensed nurse competence, potential for harm, frequency, level of decision making, and ability for self-care.

The four basic steps in delegating effectively include selecting a competent individual, explaining both the task and outcome anticipated, giving the authority and resources necessary to complete the task, and providing opportunity for input and evaluation. When trying to decide which tasks are appropriate to delegate, the following should be considered: the potential for harm, the complexity of the activity, the degree of problem solving and innovation required, the predictability of the outcome, and the extent of interaction necessary with clients. Carefully analyzing each task and matching it to an appropriate individual will assist in positive task accomplishment. The NCSBN delegation decision-making process is based on the nursing process and is in the assessment, planning, implementing, and evaluating format.

Many managers choose not to delegate because they need to control situations, fear the incompetence of their subordinates, have an attitude of superiority, or are concerned about poor outcomes. Subordinates may also be fearful of delegation because they lack self-confidence, fear criticism and overwork, have no incentives to complete new tasks, and like the convenience of having the boss solve the problems. Once a task is delegated, the delegator is still accountable for the outcome. Nurses must become familiar with the Nurse Practice Act for their state in order to understand the rules that govern nursing practice and provide direction on delegation. The American Nurses Association's Code of Ethics is a handy guide for ethical problems. Nurses must understand the liability that is inherent in delegating activities so that they can avoid any negligence through a failure to act in accordance with established standards.

Registered nurses are challenged with the delegation of tasks to unlicensed assistive personnel (UAPs). Evaluating individuals, their job description, skill level, task, and the required level of supervision they need is essential for effective delegation. Guidelines for delegating to UAP include assigning tasks that are routine and standard with outcomes that are relatively predictable and where the illness and hospitalization is not life threatening. Careful evaluation of the delegate, task, and outcome is essential for safe nursing practice. Effective use of delegation builds teams, improves an individual's skills, and enhances quality care.

Restructuring, downsizing, and redesigning initiatives have occurred in today's highly competitive marketplace. *Multiskilling* is a process where a staff member develops knowledge and takes on roles beyond those of their specialty area. Multiskilling often occurs in downsizing where one individual retains their work and in addition, takes on job duties of another role. Multiskilling is popular because employees are more productive and flexible. Nurse leaders are challenged to evaluate the staff-mix configurations in relation to cost, quality, and outcomes in patient care.

LEARNING TOOLS

Role Play #1

Delegating Tasks: Exploring Roles

Character One = Jessica is a nurse manager of a 45-bed surgical unit. Jessica is supportive of her staff and facilitates their growth and development.

Character Two = Barb is an RN on the surgical unit. She has worked for three years as an RN and is well respected by the staff. She leads a team including Julie and Anna who are both nurse's aides.

Character Three = Julie, an experienced nurse's aide on the surgical unit. She enjoys client care and works well with Barb. Julie is hesitant to offer any additional assistance to Barb even though Julie knows Barb is busy. Julie is afraid that if she offers additional assistance it will become expected of her, and she wants to leave the hospital exactly at 3:30 p.m., so she can pick her son up from school to prevent the additional expense of day care.

Character Four = Anna is a nurse's aide who was hired three months ago and has no previous experience beyond the training she has received at the hospital. Anna also feels that RNs should do more work than she does because they get paid more.

• • • • •

Barb is having trouble completing her work before the 7-3 shift ends. She feels that there is not enough time in a shift to complete the required activities for safe client care. Barb becomes frustrated when she notices the nurse's aides sitting down and chatting at the desk while she provides care at an unrelenting pace. Barb approaches Jessica explaining that she is overworked, and the nurse's aides are unproductive. She requests to have another RN put on her team. Barb tells Jessica that she would be willing to give up both nurse's aides for one experienced RN. Jessica explains to Barb that there is not enough money in the budget for any more RNs and that she will have to learn to delegate her work to the nurse's aides.

Role-Play Questions

1. What process should Barb use to determine what tasks she could delegate to Anna and Julie?
2. What should she say to Anna and Julie when she delegates tasks to them? How do you think Anna and Julie will respond?
3. Can the nurse's aides refuse to take on additional work?
4. Would both nurse's aides be able to take on the same tasks?
5. How can Barb manage the situation without becoming frustrated and burned out?

Directions: Role play this scenario showing how Julie can help Barb become comfortable with delegating. Practice delegating tasks to the nurse's aides.

Role-Play Worksheet

Characters	Student Assigned
Jessica, the nurse manager	______________
Barb, the RN	______________
Julie, the experienced nurse's aide	______________
Anna, the new nurse's aide	______________

Which character have you been assigned?

What are your character's goals in this situation?

How can the other characters assist you in achieving your goals?

What might the other characters do to hinder you in achieving your goals?

What strategies and probes do you plan to use in this situation?

CASE STUDY

Jon is an RN on the 3-11 shift for a medical unit. The nurse manager just announced that due to budget cuts, unlicensed assistive personnel (UAP) were going to be hired to assist RNs. Jon is assigned to a pod which consists of himself and two UAPs to care for 18 clients. Jon realizes he cannot complete the work himself, so he requests a description of the experience, skill level, and familiarity with the hospital of the two UAPs.

After the nurse manager provides Jon with this information, Jon goes home and identifies all the tasks that he must complete in an eight-hour shift. Based on the nurse manager's description of the UAPs' experience and skills, he assigns tasks to himself and to them. Finally, Jon develops a written mini-job description for himself and the UAPs. The next day he asks the nurse manager to review the job descriptions he has developed and asks for input. She is thrilled with the job descriptions and feels they are very appropriate. He then asks her to provide at least two hours of scheduled time for his team to get to know each other and to establish guidelines. Jon also requests one eight-hour shift when he and the two nurse's aides can have half of a normal assignment to try the new job descriptions, work out any bugs, and become comfortable with each others' expectations.

Case Study Questions

1. Is Jon using an appropriate delegation process to solve an immediate problem?
2. What are the advantages and disadvantages of the plan Jon has described?
3. What factors should Jon consider when he determines what is appropriate for delegation?

LEARNING RESOURCES

Discussion Questions

1. What are some advantages and disadvantages of delegation?
2. What is the National Council of State Boards of Nursing delegation decision-making process? How can this process be useful in practice?
3. What legal and ethical considerations do nurses who delegate tasks need to consider?

4. When a task is delegated, who then has the authority, responsibility, and accountability for the task?
5. Can all UAPs perform the same tasks? Provide a rationale for your answer.
6. Are there any tasks that managers should not delegate to their subordinates? If so, what are they, and why should they not be delegated?

Study Questions

Matching: Write the correct response in front of each term.

_____ 1. Delegator
_____ 2. Delegate
_____ 3. Supervision
_____ 4. Nursing activities
_____ 5. Non-nursing activities
_____ 6. Negligence
_____ 7. Nurse practice act
_____ 8. Board of nursing
_____ 9. ANA's Code for Nurses
_____ 10. Adaptors

A. To generate new solutions to problems
B. Failure to act in accordance with established standards
C. A source useful in exploring ethical problems
D. A set of rules that governs nursing practice
E. To function to interpret and enforce the law
F. Tasks necessary to support client care
G. Tasks necessary to provide care to clients
H. Guidance to accomplish a specific task or activity
I. The individual who accepts a new task
J. The individual who assigns a task to another

True or False: Circle the correct answer.

T F 1. Staffing patterns and methods of care delivery should be evaluated on client outcomes and basic safety.

T F 2. Multiskilling is an outdated concept that proved to be costly and unproductive in health care organizations.

T F 3. The National Council of State Boards of Nursing are opposed to delegation to unlicensed assistive personnel.

T F 4. A key element in delegation is to assess the competency level of the staff.

SUPPLEMENTAL READINGS

Bethel, S.M. (1999). Management in action. Effective leadership—six steps to productive delegating. *Clinical Laboratory Management Review, 13(3)*, 158-159.

Davidson, S.B. & Scott, R. (1999). Professional practice. Thinking critically about delegation. *American Journal of Nursing, 99(6)*, 61-62.

Fisher, M. (1999). Do your nurses delegate effectively? *Nursing Management, 30(5)*, 23-26.

Nagelkerk, J. & Henry, B. (1992-1993). Power delegating. *Graduating Nurse*, 56-57.

ANSWERS TO TEXT STUDY QUESTIONS

Chapter 12—Delegation (pp. 247–248)

1. **What does your Nurse Practice Act say about delegation and supervision?**

   Although similarities exist, each state's Nurse Practice Act has unique information concerning delegation and supervision. As a result, it is important to know the specific requisites for delegating legally and effectively in your state. You may obtain a copy of your state's Nurse Practice Act from your state board of nursing.

2. **Should a nursing student delegate work?**

   It is important for nursing students to learn and practice delegation skills. As these skills require critical thinking and advanced clinical judgment, principles of effective delegation are integrated into the final semesters of the curriculum to afford students the opportunity to practice delegation under the auspices of a supervised clinical experience.

3. **How extensively is delegating to non-RN personnel used in the work settings you have experienced?**

   In addition to thinking about how extensively delegation is used, you should also consider which tasks are delegated and in which situations delegation occurs. Do you feel that the delegation was appropriate?

4. **How comfortable are you with delegation?**

   You may be hesitant or uncomfortable delegating tasks to other people. The basis for your discomfort may be related to a belief that you could do it better or quicker yourself, a lack of confidence in your staff, a fear of taking a risk, a need to feel indispensable, inability to direct others, a fear of losing authority or anxiety about experiencing decreases in personal satisfaction.

5. **How do you delegate to assist others to develop further?**

   Delegation should be viewed as a learning opportunity. Delegating increasingly complex tasks after providing a foundation of knowledge and skills is an excellent way for delegates to grow. By providing responsible incremental growth experiences with adequate supervision will enhance job satisfaction and build team relationships.

6. **What criteria can be used to assess workers' competency?**

   The criteria used to assess competency must be preestablished and measurable, and completed within an established time frame. Before a task is delegated, the nurse should know the job description, including the type of education and training required to function in that role. The evaluation process should include whether the task was completed correctly, completely, and within the designated time frame. Supervision and evaluation should be an ongoing process with periodic review and feedback.

7. **Do these criteria differ for RNs and UAP? For nursing students?**

   Competencies for RNs differ from those for UAP. RNs are skilled in clinical judgment and complex decision making, necessitating cognitive, affective, and psychomotor competency validation. Nursing students are evaluated by the same criteria as the RN, taking into consideration their evolving level of skill and knowledge. UAP are evaluated according to the health care agency's job description and policies that dictate their level of education and skill.

8. **What routine activities can RNs delegate to others?**

   RNs can delegate tasks and procedures that are routine such as specimen collection, vital signs, bathing, and assisting with procedures. However, it is important to remember that just because it was right to delegate a task in one instance, it may not be right the next time. A thorough assessment of the client, task, and the abilities of the delegate should be completed prior to any delegation process. Also, you should never delegate components of professional nursing practice including nursing process, nursing diagnoses, clinical judgment, or interventions that require the specialized knowledge or skill of an RN.

9. **When you delegate your work, what then do you do?**

   The goal of delegation is to have others assist you in completing certain tasks or activities. An RN remains accountable and responsible and must supervise all those to whom nursing activities are delegated. The level of supervision will depend on the experience and the expertise of the delegate. Make sure that the delegate is aware of the resources that are available to assist him or her and any parameters for reporting back to you. If the individual has never completed the task before, use it as an opportunity to teach.

10. What is a safe or minimum nurse-client ratio? Does this differ from across care settings?

A safe or minimum nurse-to-client ratio will depend on the setting, shift, skill mix, acuity, and care context. It can vary from 1:1 in a perioperative or critical care setting to 1:10 or more in a nonacute care setting. The primary determinant of an appropriate staffing ratio is that nurses must be able to provide safe care and adequate supervision for care delivery. Staffing guidelines are often established by specialty nursing organizations and the Joint Commission on Accreditation of Healthcare Organizations.

11. What is a nurse really responsible for when he or she is responsible for care coordination and delivery?

The RN retains the responsibility and accountability for the provision of care to an assigned group of clients. It is the responsibility of the RN to complete the nursing process. The RN may delegate aspects of care for clients after assessing the potential for harm, the complexity of the task, the degree of problem solving needed, the predictability of the outcome, and the competency of the delegate. As the coordinator of care, the RN delegates appropriate aspects of care, but remain accountable for care delivery.

Team Building

STUDY FOCUS

The emergence of teamwork in health care organizations is imperative for the building of knowledge work teams. Knowledge work teams are small numbers of people working together that have complimentary knowledge to achieve a desired goal for which they hold themselves mutually accountable (Sorrells-Jones & Weaver, 1999). Health care delivery systems are becoming more complex, requiring multidisciplinary work teams to tackle difficult systems problems in a cost-controlled manner. In most health care environments, nursing is at the core of client care, providing around-the-clock access to health care services. As central players in the delivery of client care, nurses are expected to assume the role of team leaders, case managers, and coordinators of care. Many of the care-coordinating roles entail interdisciplinary consultation and intense group work.

A *group* is a collection of interrelated individuals working toward a goal. Group interactions are composed of five elements: process, standards, decision making, communication, and roles (Book & Galvin, 1975). *Process* is the way the group works together to accomplish goals. *Standards* are values and norms that the group uses to process information. *Decision making* is the method the group uses to solve problems. Communication includes verbal and nonverbal interactions, both within and external to the group. Roles describe each individual's part in the group. Creative techniques used by groups to enhance group process and improve outcomes include brainstorming, nominal group technique, tri-council, and the delphi survey. Characteristics of highly effective groups include having a common purpose, agreeing on performance goals, recruiting competent members, working together, developing a collaborative climate, being mutually accountable, and setting standards of excellence.

Groups progress through a series of four stages: orientation, adaptation, emergence, and working (Farley & Stoner, 1989). The orientation stage occurs at the beginning of the group's formation and involves trust and boundary issues. During adaptation, a team's identity is formed and individual roles are differentiated. In the emergence control phase, issues arise and are resolved. The working phase is the productive stage when decision making and task accomplishment take place. These stages of the group process are not necessarily sequential and may be iterative.

People join groups for a variety of reasons. Often, people seek group participation to fulfill affiliation and achievement needs. When individuals work in groups, they gain the advantage of a greater depth and breadth of knowledge and information. Also, members of groups tend to accept and endorse group solutions to problems because of their commitment and investment in the decision-making process. Complex problems are more manageable within groups because they tend to have an increased knowledge base and a varied approach to problem solving. In groups, individuals are provided with the outlet for an expression of ideas. The disadvantages of groups can include premature decision making, individual domination and control, and disruptive conflicts. Individuals will belong to groups as long as their needs are being met. Once the costs of membership become greater than the benefits, termination will likely occur. Work group disruption leads to negative outcomes (Leppa, 1996).

Much of group work is organized and completed through meetings. Meetings are typically held to disseminate information, seek opinions, and solve problems. The important components of a successful meeting are distribution of an agenda, careful selection of members, attention to starting times and seating positions, and facilitation of discussion of the issues. Committees are formally designated groups. Committees meet at scheduled times and have an identified purpose. Task forces or ad hoc committees are specially formed to respond to a pressing need. Once the need is met, the task force is disbanded.

A continuum of authority in group decision making includes the autocratic, the consultative, the joint, and the delegated styles. The leader's style of facilitating the group's decision making affects the power of the group. The leader's role is pivotal in facilitating positive work groups to accomplish organizational goals. The leader must redirect disruptive group members such as compulsive talkers, nontalkers, interrupters, squashers, and busybodies. Team building is an essential component of the group leader's role.

Work teams are forming in health care organizations as a survival mechanism. The three types of health care teams are primary work teams, executive leadership teams, and ad hoc teams. Key steps to designing highly effective health care teams include defining the work of the team, differentiating responsibilities within the pool, narrowing the options to those most attractive, and identifying the best design to implement (Manion, Lorimer, & Leander, 1996). The seven steps to implement organization-wide teams include learning about teams, conducting an organizational assessment, determining desired outcomes, conducting a feasibility study, making decisions, creating a leadership role, and establishing a design team. Four essential components of high-performance teams include having positive roles, engaging in productive activities, sustaining cohesive relationships, and building supportive environments. The success of health care organizations in developing effective and productive knowledge-based work teams will provide strategic advantages in a highly competitive turbulent environment.

LEARNING TOOLS

Group Activity: Winter Survival Decision Exercise

Purpose: To compare autocratic, consultative, joint, and delegated group decision-making authority.

1. Divide the study group into four small groups of 7 to 12. One member of each small group will be the designated leader, one member will be the designated observer, and all other members will be participants in the small group during this exercise. Group 1 should be assigned autocratic group decision authority, Group 2 should be assigned consultative group decision authority, Group 3 should be assigned joint group decision authority, and Group 4 should be assigned delegated group decision-making authority.
2. The observer should be attuned to the process by which the groups make decisions. Crucial issues are how well the group uses the resources of its members, how much commitment to implement the decision is mustered, how the future decision-making ability of the group is affected, and how members feel about and react to what is taking place. The observer should address the following issues: Who does and does not participate in discussion? Who participates most? Who participates least? Who influences the decision? Who does not influence the decision? How is influence determined (expertise, loudness)? What are the dominant group feelings? What resources are used to make a decision?
3. Give each group the following exercise and the Winter Survival Decision Form.

You have crash-landed into a lake in the northern Minnesota woods. It is 11:32 a.m. in mid-January. The pilot and copilot were killed. Shortly after the crash, the plane sinks completely into the lake with the pilot's and copilot's bodies inside. None of you are seriously injured, and you are all dry.

The crash came suddenly, before the pilot had time to radio for help or inform anyone of your position. Since your pilot was trying to avoid a storm, you know the plane was considerably off course. The pilot announced shortly before the crash that you were twenty miles northwest of a small town that is the nearest known habitation.

You are in a wilderness area made up of thick woods broken by many lakes and streams. The snow depth varies from above the ankles in windswept areas to knee-deep where it has drifted. The last weather report indicated that the temperature would reach –25 degrees F in the daytime and –40 degrees at night. Plenty of dead wood and twigs are in the immediate area. You are dressed in winter clothing appropriate for city wear — suits, pantsuits, street shoes, and overcoats.

While escaping from the plane, several members of your group salvaged twelve items. Your task is to rank these items according to their importance to your survival. You may assume that the number of passengers is the same as the number of persons in your group and that the group has agreed to stick together.

Winter Survival Decision Form

Directions: Rank the following items according to their importance to your survival, starting with 1 for the least important item and proceeding to 12 for the most important item.

_____ Ball of steel wool
_____ Newspapers (one per person)
_____ Compass
_____ Hand ax
_____ Cigarette lighter (without fluid)
_____ Loaded .45 caliber pistol
_____ Sectional air map made of plastic
_____ Twenty-by-twenty-foot piece of heavy-duty canvas
_____ Extra shirts and pants for each survivor
_____ Can of shortening
_____ Quart of 100-proof whiskey
_____ Family-size chocolate bars (one per person)

4. Provide 45 minutes for each group to work through this exercise, then ask them to score their answers.

Scoring: Score the net difference between the participants' answers and the correct answer. For example, if a participant's answer is 9 and the correct answer is 12, the net difference is 3. Disregard all plus or minus signs. Find only the net difference for each item. Total all the item scores. The lower the score the more accurate the ranking.

Winter Survival Exercise: Answer Key

Item	Expert Ranking	Your Rank	Difference Score
Ball of steel wool	2		
Newspaper (one per person)	8		
Compass	12		
Hand ax	6		
Cigarette lighter (without fluid)	1		
Loaded .45-caliber pistol	9		
Sectional air map made of plastic	11		
Twenty-by-twenty foot piece of heavy-duty canvas	5		
Extra shirt and pants for each survivor	3		
Can of shortening	4		
Quart of 100-proof whiskey	10		
Family-size chocolate bar (one per person)	7		
Total			

5. Have the observer brief the small groups with his or her observations. This is a good time to discuss effective group decision-making techniques. Provide 15 minutes for this activity.

6. Get the total group back together, and have the leader of each group share their group scores, the type of group decision-making authority that their group were role-playing, and key observations made by the observers of their small groups.

(From Johnson, D.W. & Johnson, F.P. *Joining Together: Group Theory and Group Skills*, third edition. Copyright © 1986. All rights reserved. Adapted by permission of Allyn & Bacon.)

CASE STUDY

Jackie, a nurse practitioner who works in a primary care setting, feels isolated from other nurse practitioners because there are only physician assistants and physicians where she is employed. Jackie organizes a nurse practitioner group, invites other nurse practitioners to attend, and arranges the meeting place. The first meeting is a formal organizational gathering where people introduce themselves, socialize, and become familiar with one another and the purpose for the group. Goals are set and roles are assigned at the second, third, and fourth meetings. During the next several meetings, a number of individuals try to control the issues that are to be addressed. Once the issues are determined and people agree to be responsible for tasks, the work progresses quickly, and the group feels a sense of accomplishment.

Case Study Questions

1. What stages did this group work through?
2. What are the four stages of group progress and what do they include?
3. Do groups progress sequentially through the stages?

LEARNING RESOURCES

Discussion Questions

1. What is the continuum of authority for group decision making? How does the leader's style of facilitating the group affect group decision-making authority?
2. What are the types of disruptive group members, and what are strategies to redirect their energy toward group work and goal accomplishment?
3. What are the possible roles for clinical nurses in an interdisciplinary team?
4. What is the difference between a meeting, a committee, and a task force?
5. What are the stages of group development? Provide leader strategies to facilitate the group process for each stage.
6. What are the advantages and disadvantages of group work?
7. Describe the leader's role in planning and conducting a meeting.
8. Why are knowledge-based work teams important to a health care organization's success and viability?

Study Questions

True or False: Circle the correct answer.

T F 1. Interdisciplinary work teams are necessary for complex situations.

T F 2. Groups sequentially go through the stages of orientation, adaptation, emergence, and working.

T F 3. The major reason people join groups is to gain information.

T F 4. Group decision making is cost-effective in all situations.

T F 5. A group leader must organize and structure a group for success.

T F 6. In all groups, decision making is a joint process with all members participating.

T F 7. A committee is a formally designated group designed to meet organizational objectives.

T F 8. A task force is designed to solve long-term problems.

T F 9. Team building is a complex process that requires leader and group commitment and cooperation.

T F 10. The ideal number of members in a group is between 10-14.

T F 11. A knowledge work team is a large number of highly skilled individuals with complimentary knowledge who come together to accomplish specific goals.

T F 12. In large health care organizations interdisciplinary teams are an integral part of the core structure.

T F 13. Research has linked work group disruption with increased productivity and collaboration.

T F 14. Two elements that promote efficient and effective committee decision making are appropriate representation and delegation of authority to the committee.

REFERENCES

Book, C. & Galvin, K. (1975). *Instruction in and about small group discussion*. Falls Church, VA: Speech Communication Association.

Farley, M, & Stoner, M. (1989). The nurse executive and interdisciplinary team building. *Nursing Administration Quarterly, 13(2)*, 24-30.

Leppa, C.J. (1996). Nurse relationships and work group disruption. *Journal of Nursing Administration, 26(10)*, 23-27.

Manion, J., Lorimer, W. & Leander, W.J. (1996). *Team-based health care organizations: Blueprint for success*. Gaithersburg, MD: Aspen.

Sorells-Jones, J. & Weaver, D. (1999). Knowledge workers and knowledge-intense organizations. I. A promise framework for nursing and healthcare. *Journal of Nursing Administration, 29(7/8)*, 12-18.

SUPPLEMENTAL READINGS

Blount, K. & Nahigian, E. (1998). How to build teams in the midst of change. *Nursing Management, 29(8)*, 27-29.

Gaynor, S.E., Reschak, G.L., & Verdin, J. (1994). Evaluating a committee structure. *Journal of Nursing Administration, 24(7/8)*, 59-63.

Herman, J.E. & Reichelt, P.A. (1998). Are first-line nurse managers prepared for team building? *Nursing Management, 29(10)*, 68-72.

Johnson, D.W. & Johnson, F.P. (1987). *Joining Together*. New Jersey: Prentice-Hall, Inc.

O'Connell (1999). Teams: The future of leading. *Surgical Service Management, 5(5)*, 40-2.

Wheelan, S.A. & Burchill, C. (1999). Take teamwork to new heights. *Nursing Management, 30(4)*, 28-82.

ANSWERS TO TEXT STUDY QUESTIONS

Chapter 13—Team Building (p. 271)

1. **Does nursing need to be structured into work groups for effective client care delivery?**

   In today's health care climate the coordination aspect of nursing practice is paramount, necessitating a collaborative approach to the provision of client care in work groups. The nurse serves as the central coordinator of care and must work collaboratively with multiple disciplines to effectively and efficiently provide cost-effective, quality care. The work group provides the forum for nurses and other care providers to join together to formulate client care decisions and to improve work processes.

2. **What motivates an individual to join a group?**

   An individual may join a group to satisfy psychological drives and primary needs. The need for socialization, affiliation, and recognition, as well as an opportunity for self-achievement, often motivate group participation.

3. **What are the significantly different elements between social groups and organizational groups? What elements are similar?**

   Organizational groups are established to create a sense of status and esteem, to test and establish reality, and to accomplish work. The primary elements in social groups are opportunities for interactions with people and a sense of self-achievement. Both types of groups provide opportunities for social exchange.

4. **How is leading a group like the nursing process? The management process?**

   Leading a group parallels the nursing process in that it consists of assessment, diagnosis, planning, intervention, and evaluation. Essential functions of the group leader are to assess the group's role and responsibility and to articulate its purpose. The group leader is responsible for planning functional and operational processes, facilitating group consensus, and evaluating group work. The management process is also useful in leading a group. It involves planning, diagnosing, coordinating, implementing the best solution, and evaluating and tracking outcomes. Additional components of the management process include organizing the physical environment, preparing and motivating participants for action, and facilitating the group accomplishments.

5. **What team-building strategies are used in nursing? How can this process be improved?**

   Interactive leadership, a leadership style prevalent in nursing, facilitates team building. It employs such strategies as participatory management, mutual respect, and generating trust through shared governance models. Building team cohesion and performance can be enhanced by facilitating interdisciplinary collaboration, using conflict resolution skills, forming strong alliances with top decision makers, and enhancing collaboration and coordination skills.

Budgeting

STUDY FOCUS

Budgeting and financial management are crucial skills for nurses who practice the art and science of nursing. In health care resources are scarce, reimbursement structures have changed, and organizations are seeking methods to cut costs. How then can a nurse manager justify expenses, garner new resources, and compete with other health care managers for limited dollars? A strong foundation in financial management is essential.

The first phase of the financial management process is budgeting. A *budget* is the projected plan for revenues and expenses for a specified period. *Revenue* is the income generated for services provided and expenses are the cost of producing the services. A budget is a written financial plan aimed at controlling the allocation of resources in organizations. The budget is a key aspect of the planning process that identifies funds necessary for implementing programs and services. Budgeting is a component of cost accounting and is essential for providing a roadmap and is a guide to assist individuals in successfully meeting goals.

There are seven general types of budgets (Finkler and Kovner, 1993). The *operating budget* is the plan for the daily operating revenue and expenses for a specified unit or organization for a designated period. Elements included in the operational budget include a workload budget with activity reports, units of service, and workload calculations; expense budgets for personnel, staffing requirements, and labor costs; expense budgets for supplies, equipment, and overhead; and a revenue budget. A *long-range budget* is a strategic plan that establishes goals over long periods, often 3, 5, and 10 years. A *program budget* evaluates a specific program that often involves more than one department over a period of several years. A *capital budget* tracks the purchase of large assets like buildings, land, or large costly pieces of equipment. In many organizations, a capital purchase is any item greater than $500. A *product line budget* is the revenues and expenses associated with a defined group of clients. A *cash budget* logs the cash receipts and disbursements on a monthly basis. A *special purpose budget* is developed for programs or services that were not included in the annual budget.

Familiarity with the three basic types of budgets will assist nurse managers when interacting with financial personnel. *Traditional budgets* are based on expenses for the previous year with an inflation factor added. *Zero-based budgets* require the manager to rebuild the budget each year justifying all line items. *Performance budgets* are based on the activities of a cost center.

Managers also track direct and indirect expenses. Direct costs are those items that result in providing physical care to the client. Indirect costs include overhead, supportive, and administrative expenses. Nurse managers also measure the intensity of care by examining the amount, type, and cost of nursing care for client groups.

The budgetary process involves four phases: disseminating instructions, preparing the first budget draft, reviewing and adjusting, and appealing. There are two key components of budgeting—volume and cost measures. Volume measures are activity standards based on a workload measure for the organization. The cost measure is commonly a salary standard.

Some of the largest expenses in health care organization budgets are nursing personnel and supply usage. The large size of nursing departments puts nurses at risk for layoffs and downsizing. Nurses will be called upon to contain costs and provide high-quality health care. Suggestions for nurses that promote cost control include doing a job efficiently, motivating clients to recover, using supplies carefully, and maximizing the use of time. Nurse managers may use internal and external benchmarking as a mechanism to evaluate their budgeting and staffing. Nurse managers may also cost out nursing services to determine the actual "cost" of care provided by client type. Nurses must be able to identify and charge for services provided instead of being invisible in hospital charges.

LEARNING TOOLS

Reporting Exercise

Purpose: To identify the important categories of a monthly manager's report and to identify important data for each category.

Introduction: Nurse managers have 24-hour accountability for the staffing, management, and leadership of their assigned unit(s). They are fiscally responsible and must manage their resources to stay within budget or within the adjusted budget based on client days, adjustments in acuity, and length of stay. Most managers are held accountable in four major categories: financial, material, human, and unit goals. The financial data category reflects the actual versus budgeted expenses for each line item (such as equipment, supplies, and salaries). Variances both positive and negative are reported and justified. The material data category reports changes in products or supplies, any equipment trials or examinations, and any changes in procedures for the unit(s). The human resource category reflects any concerns, issues, accomplishments, and critical incidents as well as any unit news or individual education, or professional achievement. The last column is for unit goals established by the nurse manager and reported monthly and annually. These goals may include budget variance predictions, staffing issues, or procedural changes.

Depicted below is a form that could be used to report monthly data:

Monthly Report

I. Financial Indicators: List any variances for line items and provide rationale for the positive or negative variance.

II. Material Issues: Describe any changes in materials or supplies, any equipment trials, or any changes in procedures requiring changes in materials.

III. Human Relations: Describe any concerns, critical incidents, issues, accomplishments, or personal and professional achievements.

IV. Unit Goals: Describe accomplishments toward your established unit goals and provide data on your progress.

Directions: Use the data in the following case study to complete the monthly report.

CASE STUDY

Susan is the nurse manager for a 46-bed general surgical unit in Palm Harbor, Florida. Susan has just received her revenue and expense report for the month. She has been speaking with the chief financial officer (CFO) about the possibility of receiving biweekly revenue and expense reports because she feels that problems cannot be corrected quickly with such a delay in reporting. In response, the CFO is working out the mechanics to issue reports every two weeks to help managers react more quickly to fiscal issues. (See below for revenue and expense report.) Susan is also testing new syringes on her unit, and Cam, an RN on 7-3, has streamlined the procedure for collecting and sending specimens to the laboratory. Susan has been tracking the unit's critical incidents and discovers three medication errors for the same nurse within a two-week period. Sally, an RN on 3-11 has just completed an RN-BSN program, and Ron, an RN, has just passed a certification exam. Susan's unit goals were to stay within 2% of budget; to assist nurses to continue their education through certification, continuing education, or formal education; and to analyze the activities that could be completed by nursing assistants to decrease their down time.

Cost Center: 611 General Surgery | Report For June 2000

This Month			Account	Year to Date		
Actual	Budget	Variance	Number/Description	Actual	Budget	Variance
			311. Revenue			
(371,026)	(365,800)	5,226	0110 Routine	(3,244,410)	(3,221,400)	23,010
(2,987)	(3,153)	(166)	020 Other	(27,590)	(27,768)	(178)
(374,013)	(368,953)	5,060	Total Operating Rev	(3,272,000)	(3,249,168)	22,832
			411. Salary Expense			
85,115	85,127	12	010 Salaries-Regular	730,881	749,665	18,784
2,758	0	(2,758)	020 Salaries-Per Diem	2,758	0	(2,758)
3,209	4,101	892	030 Salaries-Overtime	40,128	36,115	(4,013)
10,885	11,220	335	040 Salaries Differential	97,995	98,810	815
7,168	7,066	(102)	050 FICA	61,285	62,222	937
7,235	7,363	128	060 Health Insurance	62,125	64,846	2,721
2,212	2,358	146	070 Pension	19,855	20,766	911
1,896	1,915	19	080 Other	17,228	16,868	(360)
120,478	119,150	(1,328)	Total Salary Expense	1,032,255	1,049,292	17,037
			611. Supply Expense			
4,976	4,084	(892)	010 Patient Care Supplies	41,692	35,961	(5,731)
118	202	84	020 Office Supplies	1,097	1,780	683
371	366	(5)	030 Forms	3,111	3,224	113
0	127	127	040 Supplies Purchased	1,210	1,122	(88)
250	191	(59)	050 Equipment	1,553	1,683	130
125	149	24	060 Seminars/Meetings	1,163	1,309	146
25	17	(8)	070 Books	145	150	5
0	112	112	080 Equipment Rental	385	987	602
31	64	33	090 Miscellaneous	388	561	173
5,896	5,312	(584)	Total Supply Expense	50,744	46,777	(3,967)
			911. Interdepartmental Expense			
934	921	(13)	010 Central Supply	7,828	8,114	286
1,137	1,121	(16)	020 Pharmacy	9,527	9,868	341
1,915	1,888	(27)	030 Linen/Laundry	16,046	16,628	582
105	297	192	040 Maintenance	977	2,618	1,641
211	212	1	060 Telephone	1,962	1,870	(92)
0	21	21	070 Photocopy	124	187	63
0	13	13	090 Miscellaneous	165	112	(53)
4,302	4,473	171	Total Interdepartmental Expense	36,629	39,397	2,768
130,676	128,935	(1,741)	Total Operating Expense	1,119,628	1,135,466	15,838
(243,337)	(240,018)	3,319	Contributions from Operations	(2,152,372)	(2,113,702)	38,670
65.1%	65.1%		Contributions % of Revenue	65.8%	65.1%	

Budgeting Exercise

Introduction: It is important to have a basic understanding of budgeting and financial management as a clinical nurse. This section will provide definitions of terms, simple calculations, and answers to the calculations.

I. A unit of service is a measurement that describes an activity in an organization. The units of service are what determine the revenue or income of the organization and describe the needed resources to offer the service.

The following definitions are basic to budgeting and financial calculations:

Beds = number of beds available for occupancy
Census = number of clients occupying beds at a specific time of day (usually midnight)
Percent occupancy = census divided by beds available x 100
Patient day = one client occupying one bed for one day
Average daily census (ADC) = patient days in a given period divided by the number of days in the period
Average length of stay (ALOS) = client days in a given period divided by number of discharges in the period

(Definitions and budgeting calculations were taken from Finkler, S.A. (1992). *Budgeting Concepts for Nurse Managers*. Philadelphia: W.B. Saunders Co.)

II. How do client classification systems work? Classification systems are based on instruments that reflect critical indicators of care requirements. Based on the absence or presence of indicators, clients are assigned a score. Below is a printout of a classification.

Client Type	Required Care Hours in 24 Hours		Relative Value
	Range	Average	
1	0.5-2.9	2.0	0.4
2	3.0-6.9	5.0	1.0
3	7.0-15.4	10.0	2.0
4	15.5-24.0	22.0	4.4

In this example, the patient type is simply a descriptor of the classification categories. A Type 1 patient has the least workload requirements and a Type 4 the most. The range indicates the amount of care required, and the average is the assigned value of care for all Type 1 patients. The relative value scale puts the hours of care required for each type of patient in a workload measure. Type 2 patients are arbitrarily assigned a workload value of 1.0 taking 5 hours of care on average; and Type 3, therefore, are assigned a double workload factor because of the 10 average hours of care required.

III. How are acuity levels calculated? Listed below is a census of 18 patients with patient types identified. The calculation for acuity level is workload divided by census = acuity (24.0 divided by 18 = 1.33).

Client Type	Number of Clients	Relative Value	Workload
1	4	0.4	1.6
2	8	1.0	8.0
3	5	2.0	10.0
4	1	4.4	4.4
Total	18		24.0

What would the average acuity level be for this population? The calculation for average acuity is workload divided by census = acuity (120.0 divided by 18 = 6.67).

Client Type	Required Average in 24 Hours	Number of Clients	Workload
1	2.0	4	8.0
2	5.0	8	40.0
3	10.0	5	50.0
4	22.0	1	22.0
Total		18	120.0

Employers frequently discuss the terms FTEs (full-time equivalent employees) and positions or position control. These are common terms used to discuss the manpower needs of a unit or an organization. Most organizations hire at least 60-80% of their workforce with full-time equivalent employees. A full-time equivalent in hours per year = 2080. A full-time equivalent per week = 40 hours. Job positions that the unit/organization has or will hire are part-time, full-time, or per diem. Each unit is allocated a number of full-time and part-time positions, which is then referred to in some institutions as a position control. The position control, or number of full-time, part-time, and per diem employees, is allocated, as well as the type (registered nurse, licensed practical nurse, unlicensed assistive personnel) that they are permitted to hire to cover the workload of the unit.

LEARNING RESOURCES

Discussion Questions

1. Describe the three different types of budgets—zero-based, performance, and traditional.

2. Discuss how acuity levels are calculated and workload needs are determined.
3. What is the nurse's role in providing high-quality health care and containing costs for the organization?
4. What is the difference between an operating, long-range, program, capital, product line, cash, and special purpose budget?
5. Should nurses concern themselves with costing out nursing care? If so, why? If not, why not?

Study Questions

Matching: Write the letter of the correct response in front of each term.

_____ 1. Budget
_____ 2. Expenses
_____ 3. Strategic planning
_____ 4. Revenues
_____ 5. Cash budget
_____ 6. Capital budget
_____ 7. Expense budget
_____ 8. Indirect costs
_____ 9. Traditional budget
_____ 10. Zero-based budget

A. A form of budgeting where the whole budget is built from scratch
B. A form of budgeting where baseline data for the budget is determined from previous cost plus an inflation factor
C. Expenses related to overhead, administration, or building
D. Income for the provision of services
E. A financial plan that guides resource use
F. Costs incurred for services provided
G. Formulation of strategy for the organization
H. Indicates receipts and disbursements
I. Indicates major purchases of $500 or more
J. Indicates payment of wages, benefits, and maintenance

SUPPLEMENTAL READINGS

Brown, B. (1999). Financial management: How to develop a unit personnel budget. *Nursing Management, 30(6)*, 34-35.

Craske, C. (1997). Leadership. Cash control...controlling the budget. *Nursing Times, 93(12)*, 69-71.

Jones, K.R. (1999). Finance for nurse managers. Types of budgets. *Seminars for Nurse Managers, 7(1)*, 5-6.

Sengin, K.K. & Dreisbach, A.M. (1995). Managing with precision: A budgetary decision support model. *Journal of Nursing Administration, 25(2)*, 33-44.

Shamian, J., Hagen, B., & Fogarty, T. (1994). The relationship between length of stay and required nursing care hours. *Journal of Nursing Administration, 24(7/8)*, 52-58.

ANSWERS TO TEXT STUDY QUESTIONS

Chapter 14—Budgeting (p. 288)

1. **How does budgeting relate to leadership, control, and management in health care?**

   A budget is a written document used to forecast revenues and expenditures in order to control costs and to allocate resources. Although the development of the budget and the evaluation of its effectiveness is a managerial responsibility, staff nurse leadership is also needed to motivate other individuals to implement the financial plan and accomplish the objectives of the budget.

2. **Do nurses raise health care costs or lower them?**

   Health care agencies are the largest employers of nurses, with a large proportion of the personnel budget allocated to their salaries. Although nurses' salaries may result in substantial expenditures, nurses can reduce health care costs through responsible and well-informed clinical decision making, efficient care provision, and astute resource management. Without constant attention to these details by nurses, health care costs will escalate.

3. **How would a nurse manager manage a revenue budget?**

   Operating revenues are calculated by multiplying the services provided by the charges for the services. Nurse managers can manage the revenue budget by making sure that all services are charged for, that all charges are appropriate, that reimbursement is maximized, and that new methods to increase revenue are investigated.

4. **What leadership roles and activities are important in budgeting?**

   Creative leadership is needed to justify, secure, and allocate scarce resources; influence employees to find innovative ways to work efficiently and effectively; and to explore creative resource venues. Leaders model cost-conscious behaviors, analyze expenditures, and mentor employees to facilitate financial goal attainment.

5. **What activities of budgeting are appropriate at the staff nurse level?**

   Appropriate budgeting activities for nurses include providing information concerning equipment requests, supply usage, and product evaluation. By knowing the costs of supplies, nurses can carefully select cost-effective materials, substituting less expensive items as appropriate. Budget conscious nurses can decrease the length of hospitalization by motivating clients toward recovery, minimizing scheduling errors, and encouraging interdisciplinary collaboration to optimize positive patient outcomes.

6. **How can staff nurses best acquire knowledge and skills in budgeting?**

   Nurses acquire valuable knowledge and skills from leaders that take the time to educate their staff about the budgeting process. Further knowledge is gained as nurse leaders model fiscally responsible behaviors and provide opportunities to learn budgeting skills. Participation in committees, quality improvement programs, continuing education, and college courses are other sources for gaining valuable knowledge about budgeting.

7. **How is budgeting like balancing a personal checkbook?**

   Consider your personal checkbook as your budget, reflecting your personal financial plan. You have predetermined deposits (revenues) and you write checks to cover your expenses (expenditures). How you manage your account will determine if you will maintain a positive balance. Planning, organizing, acquiring, and controlling money and resources are essential elements that are inherent in personal and organizational budgeting.

Change Management

STUDY FOCUS

Dramatic change is occurring in society creating a transition from an industrial society to an information society. The perspectives on change—making something different—are both positive and negative. Even when change is positive it can create tensions and anxiety. *Change* is a process that is inevitable in our personal and professional lives. Change ranges on a continuum from haphazard to planned. *Planned change* is intentional intervention. A *change agent* is an individual who may be used to assist with planning and implementing change. The three strategies for organizational change are the rational-empirical, the normative-reeducative, and the power-coercive. The four areas in which organizational change may occur in nursing today include the organizational structures, nursing shortage cycles, reimbursement, and information systems. Change has been described by nursing leaders as a ruthless force capable of destroying those who refuse to adapt (O'Malley, 1995).

In the United States, there have been cycles of shortages and surpluses in nursing. The nursing shortage cycles are influenced by historical, economic, and social changes. Stability in nursing and long-term growth is difficult to achieve in when there are cyclic demands for nurses. Basis of the nursing cycles are the nature of the work, low wages, poor working conditions, and hospital administrator's desire to control nursing costs and salaries. Nurses will be in increased demand as the population ages and chronic illnesses increase.

Part of planning change is examining the situational elements of organizational structure, people, and resources before implementing a change strategy. Four influences on change are individuals, face-to-face groups, organizations, and communities. Many theories can be used to facilitate the change process. The most widely used theory is Lewin's change theory. Lewin provides a framework from which a force field analysis is conducted. The three elements of his theory are unfreezing, moving, and refreezing. Unfreezing, a process in which individuals become ready to change, occurs first. During the unfreezing process, individuals become aware of unmet expectations and feel discomfort over action or inaction causing them to remove obstacles to change. The second stage is moving, which is when cognitive redefinition occurs. During the moving phase, a pretrial or testing occurs. The final stage, refreezing, is when the change occurs and is integrated and stabilized. During refreezing, leaders provide positive feedback, encouragement, and motivation to reinforce the new change.

There are many other change theories including Rogers', who proposed that both the background of the individuals and the environment are antecedents to change. Rogers identified five phases of the change process—awareness, interest, evaluation, trial, and adoption. He believes that individuals choose one of two outcomes. They either accept and adopt the change, or they reject it. Another theory is Lippitt's who expanded Lewin's work by describing seven phases of change—diagnosing the problem, assessing motivation and the capacity to change, assessing motivation and resources, selecting change objectives, choosing roles for change agents, maintaining change, and terminating the helping relationship with the change agent.

Individuals respond differently to change. Some individuals are exhilarated while others are depressed, confused, and angry. Being aware of the emotional responses to a change can assist leaders to manage and facilitate change in a positive manner. Perlman and Takas (1990) identified the ten stages of the emotional voyage during change. The ten stages are equilibrium, denial, anger, bargaining, chaos, depression, resignation, openness, readiness, and reemergence. Resistance is another important characteristic of individuals experiencing the change process. Resistance occurs for many different reasons. Some individuals are afraid of disorder and the interruption of their daily routine, while others are fearful of losing their job, power, or resources. Resistance can be useful if structured positively. Encouraging individuals to discuss change openly and to identify opportunities and barriers can create a smooth transition.

Implementing change strategies effectively leads to positive outcomes. Effective leaders have good diagnostic skills and the ability to adapt the leadership style to the situation and change some or all of the situational variables during the change process. Action steps to maintain momentum include emphasizing managerial support, answering questions and personal concerns, and exercising tolerance. Smith's (1996) change management principles include keeping performance results the prime objective, increasing the numbers of individuals involved, ensuring individuals know why their performance matters, learning by doing, embracing improvisation, using team performance, concentrating designs on the work people do, focusing energy and meaningful language, sustaining behavior-driven change, and practicing leadership based on the new changes. Seven categories of change strategies include educational, facilitative, technostructural, data-based, communication, persuasive, and coercive.

Innovations are the creation of something new. Innovation often entails a systematic, purposeful, and organized search for solutions to existing problems. Careful analysis and research occur prior to innovation. Sources of innovation include the following: examining the unexpected, incongruity, process needs, changes in industry or market structure, demographics, new knowledge, and change in perceptions or moods (Drucker 1992). McCloskey, et al. (1994) identified five types of nursing innovations: introducing new technology, creating personnel development strategies, changing the organization of work, changing rewards/incentives, and implementing quality improvement mechanisms.

Strong leadership in nursing is needed to be proactive to the continuous learning and adapting required in an era of unprecedented change. Transformational change ignites passion in people, creativity and encourages innovations. Health care is in a paradigm shift. The transformations in health care include focus on the population as customer, wellness care, cost management, interdependence, quality information to consumer, and continuity of information. Investing in people's innovations, creativity, and nontraditional solutions provides strategic advantages in health care.

LEARNING TOOLS

Activity

Purpose: To examine and use a change theory evaluation instrument to assess the utility of a specific change theory for your desired change.

Introduction: Change is inevitable, occurring continuously in our daily lives. By taking charge of change and planning change activities, you can maintain control over a turbulent environment. Many change theories are in the literature. By evaluating the theory you wish to use with a specific planned change, you will have a clear sense of the utility of the change theory for your desired change. The following tool will assist you with evaluating change theories.

Identify a pet project that you would like to institute at work. Select a planned change theory that you would like to use to assess the readiness for the change, guide the process of change, and assist you at the evaluation of the change. Huber text pp. 15-8 through 15-13 describes several change theories. Use the Tiffany/Lutjens Planned Change Theory Evaluation Instrument to assess the utility of the change theory for your pet project.

The Tiffany/Lutjens Planned Change Theory Evaluation Instrument

The scoring for this tool is 0 for "I fully disagree" to 4 for "I fully agree."

Directions: Choose a change theory. Write a number from 0 to 4 on the line in front of the statement that reflects your beliefs about the utility of this theory to your specific change.

I. Significance

_____ 1. The planned change theory addresses targets for change.

_____ 2. This theory has an assessment process that could help a change agent identify a problem in a social system.

_____ 3. The theory has a clear process for evaluating the total change event.

_____ 4. The theory accounts for emerging problems and/or goals throughout the change process.

_____ 5. The theory prompts nursing change agents to ask if the proposed change is important for nursing.

_____ 6. The theory encourages the ethical use of power.

_____ 7. The theory encourages close cooperation between change agents and target populations.

_____ 8. The theory encourages change agents to help people in the target population make informed decisions.

_____ 9. The theory stresses social justice.

_____ 10. The theory looks at the world as a whole.

_____ 11. The theory views the world as changing rather than nonchanging.

_____ 12. The theory prompts change agents to consider whether the strategies they plan will agree with expectations of the social unit targeted for change.

II. Clarity and Consistency

_____ 13. This theory has a clear process for planning change.

_____ 14. This theory has a clear process for implementing change (causing change to occur).

_____ 15. This theory clearly defines planned change.

_____ 16. The definition of planned change fits with the remainder of the content of the theory.

_____ 17. Key ideas are clearly defined.

_____ 18. Relational statements are clearly stated.

_____ 19. Key ideas and relational statements avoid unnecessary repetition.

_____ 20. Key ideas are consistently used as defined throughout the theory.

_____ 21. The theory clearly states what it accepts as truth (assumptions).

_____ 22. Key ideas are related to one another.

_____ 23. Any diagrams offered increase the reader's understanding of planned change and its processes.

_____ 24. The planned change theory contributes to an understanding of planned change beyond what could be obtained from everyday experience or formal study of other planned change theories.

III. Generality

_____ 25. The planned change theory could help agents plan change.

_____ 26. The theory focuses only on the processes of planned change, not on unplanned change.

_____ 27. The purpose of the theory allows a change agent to carry out plans for change in any one of a number of clinical settings rather than in one specific setting or area.

_____ 28. This theory could apply to individuals.

_____ 29. This theory could apply to groups.

_____ 30. This theory could apply to communities.

_____ 31. This theory could apply to society.

_____ 32. This theory could apply to different cultures both within and outside the United States.

_____ 33. Nurses could use this theory as a foundation for research.

_____ 34. The theory could be tested through research.

_____ 35. Hypotheses that can be tested could be developed from the theory.

_____ 36. Key ideas and processes of the theory can be observed in the real world.

IV. Practicality

_____ 37. The theory prompts change agents to consider time frames.

_____ 38. The theory prompts change agents to consider the people (including experts) available to make the change.

_____ 39. The theory prompts change agents to consider space, equipment, and supplies.

_____ 40. The theory prompts change agents to consider financial resources.

_____ 41. The theory prompts change agents to consider organizational support.

_____ 42. The theory promotes change agents to consider whether they can obtain needed political resources for implementing change.

_____ 43. The theory prompts change agents to consider whether they can obtain needed legal resources for implementing change.

V. Applicability

_____ 44. Nurse change agents could use this theory to create change in clinical settings.

_____ 45. Nurse change agents could use this theory to create change in nursing education.

_____ 46. Nurse change agents could use this theory to create change in nursing administration.

VI. Foresight

_____ 47. The theory helps change agents to foresee possible procedural pitfalls in planning change.

_____ 48. The theory helps change agents to foresee possible cultural pitfalls in planning change.

_____ 49. The theory suggests ways to deal with possible procedural pitfalls in planning change.

_____ 50. The theory suggests ways to deal with possible cultural pitfalls in planning change.

_____ 51. The theory helps change agents to foresee immediate resistance to change.

_____ 52. The theory helps change agents to foresee long-term resistance to change.

_____ 53. The theory helps change agents to foresee the immediate results of adopting the proposed solutions.

_____ 54. The theory helps change agents to foresee the long-term results of adopting the proposed solutions.

Scoring: This tool helps you to see how well the change theory fits your specific change situation. As you score the statements, you are able to tell how well the theory meets your change process needs. Overall, the higher the total score (adding up each number for all 54 items = highest total score, 216), the better the fit between the change theory and your change situation.

CASE STUDY

Evelyn, a nurse manager of a 47-bed oncology unit in a large teaching hospital in Cincinnati, Ohio, decides to implement a new system of shift reporting because the current system is too lengthy. She first introduces the idea at a staff meeting and discusses several different options as well as the problems with the current system. She discusses the difficulties of providing high-quality client care for the first 45 minutes of each shift. Evelyn then opens the meeting for discussion. She encourages both objections and support for each idea. Evelyn elicits volunteers to work on the planned change. After two months, Evelyn asks the task force to report back their findings and propose a new method for the reporting structure for the unit. Individuals are again encouraged to both critique and support the proposal. After this meeting, modifications in the new reporting format are made and the plan is implemented. Evelyn and the task force make a point to reinforce the change with the staff and to provide them with encouragement and support when any difficulties arise.

Case Study Questions

1. Did Evelyn use a change theory? If so, which one?
2. What steps of the change theory do you see in this case study?
3. Why did Evelyn and the task force encourage the staff to raise concerns and verbalize resistance?

LEARNING RESOURCES

Discussion Questions

1. Discuss the similarities and differences of Lippitt's and Rogers' change theories.
2. What is an innovation? Discuss nursing innovations with which you are familiar.
3. Discuss potential emotional responses to change, and describe how you would facilitate the change process when encountering these responses.
4. What are four major changes occurring in the health care industry today? What are some strategies to manage these changes effectively?
5. How can resistance positively affect change? What should a leader do when resistance is encountered?

Study Questions

True or False: Circle the correct answer.

T F 1. Change is inevitable and is necessary for organizational viability.

T F 2. Resistance can be useful and should be listened to and analyzed.

T F 3. Lippitt's change theory involves the phases of unfreezing, moving, and refreezing.

T F 4. Change is a linear process requiring a series of discrete steps.

T F 5. Resistance most commonly arises because individuals are trying to gain more power.

T F 6. Changing individual behavior requires considerable time and energy.

T F 7. Individuals become aware of the need for change when needs are unmet.

T F 8. Position power can be used effectively to initiate change.

T F 9. Change occurs in a logical, planned manner.

T F 10. Too much change is disruptive and can create disorganization.

REFERENCES

Drucker, P. (1992). *Managing for the Future: The 1990s and Beyond.* New York: Truman Talley Books/Plume.

McCloskey, J., Maas, M., Huber, D., Kasparek, A., Specht, J., Ramler, C., Watson, C., Blegen, M., Delaney, C., Ellerbe, S., Estscheidt, C., Congaware, C., Johnson, M., Kelley, K., Mehmert, P. & Clougherty, J. (1994). Nursing management innovations: a need for systematic evaluation. *Nursing Economic$, 12(1)*, 35-44.

Perlman, D. & Takacs, G. (1990). The 10 stages of change. *Nursing Management, 21(4)*, 33-38.

Smith, D.K. (1996). *Taking charge of change: 10 principles for managing people and performance*. Reading, MA: Addison-Wesley.

SUPPLEMENTAL READINGS

Davidhizar, R., Shearer, R. & Dowd, S.B. (1999). When the nurse manager must help staff cope with change. *Seminars for Nurse Managers, 7(2)*, 81-85.

Moulding, N.T., Silagy, C.A. & Weller, D.P. (1999). A framework for effective management of change in clinical practice: Dissemination and implementation of clinical practice guidelines. *Quality in Health Care, 8(9903)*, 177.

Murphy, S. (1999). Mindshift for managers: Change is inevitable, growth is optimal. *Home Health Care Management & Practice, 11(2)*, 6-14.

South, S.F. (1999). Managing change isn't good enough. *Clinical Laboratory Management Review, 13(1)*, 22-26.

Tiffany, C.R., Cheatham, A.B., Doornbos, D., Loudermelt, L. & Momadi, G.G. (1994). Planned change theory: Survey of nursing periodical literature. *Nursing Management, 25(7)*, 54-59.

ANSWERS TO TEXT STUDY QUESTIONS

Chapter 15—Change Management (p. 309)

1. **How do individuals in organizations get the information resources that they need to effect change?**

   Individuals in organizations get the information needed to effect change through regulatory agencies, legislative mandates, professional organizations, scientific investigations, and collegial networks. With an organization, information may be disseminated through formal channels of communication or through informal networks known as "grapevines."

2. **How can informal leaders be used for successful change?**

   The successful implementation of a change process cannot be achieved solely by management or formal leaders. Informal leaders can be valuable assets to the change process in that they are able to enlist the support of their contemporaries. The active participation of informal leaders can promote acceptance to change while minimizing resistance.

3. **What changes need to take place in nursing? Why?**

   Several changes need to take place in nursing. First, nursing must present itself as a profession based on a solid body of knowledge. Clinical judgments made by nurses are rooted in science and involve the diagnosis and treatment of human responses. The development of and accessibility to large databases will promote collaborative scholarly activity that will impact nursing practice and patient care. Second, nurses must be politically and socially active if they are to have control over professional practice and input into the delivery of quality patient care. Proactive efforts aimed at advancing the professional and financial status of nursing may serve as a catalyst to recruit more individuals into nursing and to deter others from leaving its ranks.

4. **How does resistance manifest itself?**

   Resistance may manifest itself in several ways. It may present in the form of frustration, aggression, or even indifference. However, resistance may belie fears such as loss of employment, power, or control. Misunderstanding the purpose and need of the change combined with the dissemination of inaccurate information may serve to escalate resistance and thwart efforts necessary for the successful enactment of change.

5. **How can nurses' perceptions be changed to result in empowerment? Why is this important?**

   Nurses must be active participants in the change process. Allowing feelings and fears to be aired allows for dialogue and the exchange of ideas, while fostering autonomy and creativity. Through this process nurses will perceive their input as valuable. Individuals who feel empowered are more apt to enact changes that challenge the status quo.

6. **How should nursing education change? Why?**

   Nursing education must prepare nurses with the leadership skills necessary to initiate and enact change. Nurses must be prepared with the leadership skills necessary to interact with others, resolve conflicts, and to promote collegial relationships to build consensus and enact change. By educating novice nurses in this manner, the profession of nursing will be able to proactively and creativity take advantage of opportunities to effect changes that will improve nursing care, professional practice, and service delivery.

7. **Do we have too much change? What can be done about this?**

   Change is inevitable. It is a constant process that can be planned or unplanned. Unplanned change may precipitate feelings of fear or loss of control. However, if one can move along the continuum from haphazard to planned change, feelings of control are regained as individuals plan, examine, and adapt to the impending change. Providing information, open communication, and the active involvement of the participants supports a sense of control necessary to adapt to and accept change.

Staff Selection and Development

STUDY FOCUS

Employees are the greatest asset of a health care organization and the success of the organization depends on employee performance. Nurses are knowledge workers who provide services based on specialized knowledge and complex decision making. In a knowledge-based business, the investment in human resources is critical to organizational renewal and survival. In attracting the best and the brightest employees, career and staff development programs can be an important benefit. The process of staff selection and development are key human resource strategies for attracting the best employees.

A *human resource* is an individual employed by the organization (Jernigan, 1988). *Performance management* is an interactive process between the work that an individual accomplishes and the performance rewards and incentives provided by the organization (Frank, 1998). *Staff selection* is the process of choosing the most qualified person for a job (Jernigan, 1988). *Staff development* is the process of orientation, in-service education, and continuing education to promote the development of personnel in an employment setting. *Orientation* is the introduction of new staff to the philosophy, goals, policies, procedures, services, and facilities of the organization. *In-service education* is a learning experience provided in the work setting to assist staff to perform assigned functions (ANA, 1990). *Continuing education* involves programs that include nursing content that builds upon previously acquired knowledge and skills (ANA, 1990).

The goal of human resource development is to foster an organizational culture that makes work and the work environment positive and fulfilling. The functions of human resource management encompass job analysis, organizational development, staffing, employee relations, and evaluation (Frank, 1998). The eight personnel processes related to human resource management include recruitment, selection, orientation, performance evaluation, counseling and coaching, retention and productivity, staff development, and labor relations (Jernigan, 1988). A comprehensive integrated personnel system is detailed, behavior-oriented, and job specific, integrating the selection process, staff development, performance appraisal, and reward system.

The selection of the most qualified employee for the posted position should be based on a thorough organizational process that begins with job analysis. *Job analysis* is the evaluation of a job performed within the organization and the construction of a process for selecting employees. Job analysis data is used to develop job classification procedures, to screen applicants for vacant positions, to complete performance appraisals, and to conduct staff development and training. Employee selection is governed by regulation that guides employment practices. The United States Equal Employment Opportunity Commission (EEOC) and most other federal and state organizations require nondiscriminatory employment practices. Potential pitfalls of interviewing include excluding applicants with nonmajority attributes, not measuring occupational qualifications, and not enhancing the predictability of performance.

The job description is the base for which the interviews and hiring process originates. Thorough preparation with preplanned outlines or guides and the use of open-ended questions as prompts are effective tools for interviewing potential employees. Questions that may not be asked include marital status, children, limitation or disability, religious affiliation, alcohol or drug use, and social organization membership. Questions that may be asked include any problems with the job hours, status of United States citizenship or resident alien with the right to work, and whether the applicant can perform the essential job functions required for the position.

The primary task of nursing staff development is to provide structure and assistance to employees to refine or gain knowledge and skills in nursing practice to implement within the employing organization. The major staff development activities include orientation, in-service, competency testing, and promoting lifelong learning among staff. Often, organizations will pay for required educational programs for employees such as credentials (e.g., ACLS), programs to meet regulatory requirements, training for new equipment, and skill competency validation. Orientation programs provide new employees with theoretical and skill preparation. The orientation process is important in developing a cohesive, trusting environment that motivates employees to work collaboratively and fulfill the mission of the organization. Various strategies may be used for orientation programs and include self-directed learning modules, peer group support, preceptorships, competency-based education, small-group work, role modeling, and performance-based evaluation.

Competence is the ability to perform job functions, whereas competency is the actual performance of an individual in a given situation. Job descriptions form the basis for competence assessment. Competence assessment is performed in three domains: cognitive, affective, and psychomotor. Tools for assessing competence include patient satisfaction scores, infection control reports, peer review of psychomotor skills, and unusual occurrence reports. The Joint Commission on Accreditation of Healthcare Organizations (JCAHO) publishes a nursing care standard that calls for all nursing staff to be competent. JCAHO evaluates organizations on the development and implementation of a systematic approach to staff education, a systematic method of competency assessment, and a mechanism for orientation and education.

Effective nurse executives and managers devote considerable time, energy, and resources to developing and implementing quality human resource management systems and processes as an essential long-term investment in positive personnel outcomes. With the cycles in nursing of shortages and surpluses of registered nurses, marginal organizations react to cyclic trends instead of being proactive and maintaining strong staff selection and development programs. Hiring the right people in key positions is critical to the success or organizations. In the 1990s, nurses were being laid off and organizations were downsizing, but by 1998 a shortage of specialized registered nurses had occurred. The average pay for registered nurses in 1997 was $40,365 and for nurse practitioners $62,000 (*Nursing Needs*, 1999). Recruiting and selecting the best person for the position is critical in organizations as the cost of orientation for new employees ranges from $8,000 to $50,000 (Messmer, Abelleria & Erb, 1995).

LEARNING TOOLS

Activity

Purpose: To use and evaluate the components of an interview tool used in staff selection.

Directions: First, review the interview tool to determine the information requested of the applicant. Determine the purpose of the questions posed in the interview tool. What type of information is each question attempting to elicit?

Second, answer each question on the interview tool. This activity may be used for preparing for the interview process.

Third, partner with a colleague and ask the person the questions on the interview tool and then provide feedback. When finished with the process, reverse roles and have a colleague ask the interview questions to you and provide feedback to you.

Preparing for the Interview

1. Wear appropriate clothing—conservative, not too tight or baggy.
2. Review and answer potential interview questions.
3. Schedule an interview time when you will not be rushed—don't be late.
4. Develop a list of questions to ask the potential employer.
5. Obtain information on the unit in advance.
6. Be organized.
7. Anticipate and be prepared to interview with several individuals and in a group setting.
8. First impressions are important. Have a strong handshake, smile, establish eye contact, and address each individual by name.

Structured Interview Guide

1. What are your strongest skills? What are growth areas for you?
2. What motivates and/or rewards you?
3. Describe a situation in which you were able to positively influence the actions of others in a desired direction.
4. If a situation developed where you perceived that communication was ineffective, what steps would you implement to improve the level of communication?
5. What kinds of deadlines do you have in your current position? How do you meet them?

6. Give an example of an important goal you have set in the past and your success in reaching the goal.
7. Describe a situation when you have several things going on all at once and all seemed to be high priority. How did you manage and organize your time?
8. Describe a time when many changes were occurring simultaneously. How did you deal with all the changes?
9. Describe to us a situation you've encountered where "old solutions" didn't work and you were instrumental in implementing "new solutions."
10. Give us an example of a time in which you had to go outside of your normal process or procedure to solve a problem. What did you do and why?
11. Tell about a time in which you had to be relatively quick in coming to a decision.
12. What is the most difficult and challenging decision you have made recently? Please describe the situation.
13. Describe the most creative or innovative work project you have completed.
14. What stresses you out at work? What do you do to reduce your stress level?
15. Describe what the word "teamwork" means to you.
16. Tell us about teams you have worked on. Was the team successful? What made it that way?
17. Describe a time when you helped a peer to meet a goal or deadline.
18. What would your coworkers say about you? How important is that to you?
19. Tell us about a time in which you positively dealt with a negative situation and influenced the actions of others.
20. Describe a time when you were not in agreement with a team decision. What was the decision and why didn't you buy into it?
21. Tell us about a time when you and a peer disagreed on an issue. What happened? What did you do to resolve the situation?
22. Tell us about a change in management that was unsettling to you. Why?
23. What do you bring to this position that makes you the most qualified candidate?
24. What, if anything, concerns you about this position?
25. What questions do you have for us?

This interview guide was developed by Jeanne Roode, RN, MSN, CNA, Director of Neuroscience Services for Spectrum Health, Grand Rapids, MI.

CASE STUDY

Pat, the director of nursing staff development in a large teaching hospital in Pittsburgh, Pennsylvania, has received the final budget from central administration that is 20% less than she received the year prior. The chief executive officer, Jim, is very concerned about meeting budgetary projections, as reimbursements for services have stayed relatively constant over the past two years. Jim would like to maintain current staff and prevent a layoff by cutting costs in other areas such as staff development, freezing salaries for one year, and only purchasing essential equipment. Jim has met with all employees through open forums and discussed these issues as well as requested each employee's assistance with being innovative and providing quality services to clients.

Pat understands the need to cut costs, but now is faced with determining what services she can provide. She has employee fire safety, CPR, biohazardous waste disposal, licensure documentation, staff development activities, recruitment and retention plans, in-servicing on new equipment, and scholarships toward continuing education and college courses that pertain to employment. Pat is committed to providing integrated human resource management services.

Case Study Questions

1. How should Pat approach the problem of what activities will need to be cut or revised in light of the 20% cut in the staff development budget?
2. Who should Pat include in the decision making regarding what activities or scholarships should be cut?
3. What activities or programs must Pat keep in order to meet accreditation or regulatory requirements?
4. What activities are important to maintain and enhance staff knowledge and skills?
5. What are the major staff development activities and how should they be prioritized?

LEARNING RESOURCES

Discussion Questions

1. What is the goal of human resource development? What are the functions of human resource management?
2. What are the eight personnel processes related to human resource management in nursing?
3. What is job analysis data used for in health care organizations?
4. What is the primary task and major staff development activities?
5. How do accreditation agencies influence human resource management in organizations?

6. What are innovative methods in the implementation of human resource management programs?

STUDY QUESTIONS

Matching: Write the letter of the correct response in front of each term

_____ 1. Human resource
_____ 2. Performance management
_____ 3. Staff selection
_____ 4. Staff development
_____ 5. Orientation
_____ 6. In-service education
_____ 7. Continuing education
_____ 8. Competence
_____ 9. Competency
_____ 10. Job analysis

A. Evaluation of the position and use of the information to construct a process for employee selection
B. The process of choosing the most qualified candidate for a position
C. An individual's actual performance in a specific situation
D. An individual employed by the organization
E. The process of orientation, in-service education, and continuing education to promote the development of personnel
F. An individual's capacity to perform job functions
G. Introducing new employees to the philosophy, goals, policies, procedures, and expectations of the organization
H. Educational programs that consist of nursing knowledge that builds upon previous skills
I. Learning experiences provided in the work setting that assist employees in completing assigned functions
J. An interactive process between employee work motivation and performance rewards

REFERENCES

American Nurses Association (ANA). (1990). *Standards for nursing staff development*. Kansas City, MO: Author.

Frank, B. (1998). Performance management. In J.A. Dinemann (Ed.), *Nursing Administration: Managing Patient Care* (2nd Ed., pp. 461-484). Stamford, CT: Appleton & Lange.

Jernigan, D.K. (1988). *Human resource management in nursing*. Norwalk. CT: Appleton & Lange.

Messmer, P.R., Abelleria, A. & Erb, P. (1995). Code 50: An orientation matrix to track orientation cost. *Journal of Nursing Staff Development, 11(5)*, 261-264.

Nursing needs. (1999). *Hospitals and Health Networks, 73(7)*, 58.

SUPPLEMENTAL READINGS

Anderson, P. & Pulich, M.A. (1997). Team-based participation in the hiring process. *Health Care Supervisor, 15(4)*, 69-76.

Bania, K. & Bergmooser, G. (1997). A tool for improving supplemental staffing. *Nursing Management, 28(5)*, 78.

Flannery, T.P. & Grace, J.L. (1999). Managing nursing assets: A primer on maximizing investment in people. *Nursing Administration Quarterly, 23(4)*, 35-46.

Letizia, M. & Jennrich, J. (1998). A review of preceptorship in undergraduate nursing education: Implications for staff development. *Journal of Continuing Education, 29(5)*, 211-216.

Vandewater, D.A. & White, L. (1998). Nurse manager selection process (part 1). Survey of selection process (part 2). *Canadian Journal of Nursing Administration, 11(1)*, 65-84.

ANSWERS TO TEXT STUDY QUESTIONS

Chapter 16—Staff Selection and Development (p. 323)

1. **How do human resource management and staff development differ?**

   Human resource management is a comprehensive, integrated process used to develop a culture that maximizes employee motivation, satisfaction, longevity, and performance. While staff development is concerned with all the facets of human resource management, in nursing it is aimed at enhancing practice through orientation, competency testing, and lifelong learning.

2. **What, if any, human resource functions need to be kept within a department of nursing? Why?**

   As nursing is a knowledge-based profession that regulates its own practice, it is important to keep the human resource functions of job analysis, staffing, and performance evaluation within a department of nursing. It is imperative that knowledgeable nurse leaders who understand the scope of professional practice select competent individuals, evaluate performance, and promote professional development in order to maximize patient outcomes.

3. **How much scarce resources should be devoted to human resource management? Staff development?**

   Although human resource management and staff development may be initially expensive, both processes should be viewed as an investment that saves scarce resources in the future. Retaining competent employees enhances organizational effectiveness, reduces personnel costs for recruitment and training of new employees, and increases institutional morale and job satisfaction.

4. **How do nurses prove their competence?**

   Competencies confirm that an individual has the knowledge, skill, and ability necessary to provide care. Initially, nurses prove this competence through licensure. Subsequent validation of cognitive, affective, and psychomotor competencies occurs through competency assessment, performance appraisal, documented continuing education and workshops, and certification examinations.

5. **How much responsibility for continuing education, especially in costs, does the employer have? Should they have?**

   Although employers are fiscally responsible for providing required educational programs such as orientation, mandatory safety, and product training, they are not obligated to pay for continuing education. Yet, health care organizations have an obligation to the public to recruit and maintain competent employees. Therefore, employers should encourage and financially support continuing education endeavors to safeguard the public's trust and to recognize the value of nurses as employees with lifelong learning needs.

Performance Appraisal

STUDY FOCUS

Managing people to effectively attain a customer-responsive, high-performance organization is essential in gaining a competitive advantage through the mobilization of superior human resources. Performance is achieving organizational and social objectives and responsibilities (Hersey, Blanchard & Johnson, 1996). In organizations, performance appraisals occur in a hierarchical fashion. At the individual level, performance is measured by appraisals. At the unit level, performance is measured by budget and quality criteria. At the organizational level, performance is evaluated by accreditation agencies.

Performance management is an interactive process among performance appraisal, work motivation, and performance rewards. Performance management has three components. The three components include performance planning, coaching to reinforce and develop, and formal performance review (Hersey, Blanchard & Johnson, 1996). Performance appraisal is an integral component of performance management in health care organizations. There are four integral components of a comprehensive performance appraisal system: determining the ability required (job description), matching abilities of the employer with job requirements (personnel selection), improving employee's abilities (staff development), and enhancing employees' motivation (staff development and the reward system) (Nauright, 1987).

Performance appraisals are important in managing the quality, efficiency, and effectiveness in the provision of nursing services. Consumers and regulatory agencies are looking for assurances that practitioners are competent to provide client services within their scope of practice. One method of evaluating the practice or work of an employee is through annual performance appraisals. A *conventional performance appraisal* is a systematic standardized evaluation of an employee by a superior for the purpose of evaluating quality, effectiveness, and potential for advancement. Employer evaluation is often conducted from multiple perspectives by using peer- and self-evaluation to provide an enhanced description of individual quality and competence. Peer review consists of written or verbal input by those peers who work with the employee being evaluated into the performance appraisal. These are peers who are knowledgeable about the employee's level of performance. The goal of performance appraisals is to improve performance.

Typically, individuals' performances combine their ability and their motivation. Ability is either innate or acquired through learning, and motivation is the willingness and desire to perform work. Employees may become discouraged and lack motivation when it is punishing to complete work, when nonperformance is rewarded, when the quality of performance makes no difference, and when there are barriers to performance. Some components of evaluation are subjective, such as an evaluator's value system and expectations, and these influence the rating of an employee.

The goals of a comprehensive appraisal system include fulfilling the job description requirements, improving on employees' skills, rewarding employee motivation, and matching the right employees with the right job. Evaluations are based on standards. Absolute standards are the evaluator's personal expectations of employees based on values and knowledge. A *comparative standard* is a measurement system in which employees are compared to one another and ranked accordingly. The steps in the appraisal process include assessing and evaluating organizational needs, establishing organizational goals with specific time frames, and assessing and evaluating employee progress. In many organizations, performance assessment is continual and aimed at educating employees through coaching; through counseling to improve skills; and through ongoing, nonthreatening evaluation.

The job description and performance appraisal tools are documents that employees can use as guides to management's values. Performance appraisals improve performance and communication, reinforce positive behavior, provide rewards, document reasons for termination, and assist individuals with learning needs. Ten research-based principles for performance appraisal are rewarding and developing subordinates, training managers in evaluation, basing evaluation on job descriptions, involving employees in the evaluation, setting mutually agreed-upon goals, focusing on problem solving, separating evaluation from counseling, providing administrative support, matching job expectations with evaluation, and generating useful data for administrative decisions.

There are many performance measurement tools to evaluate performance including anecdotal notes, open-ended essays, checklists, rating scales, and behaviorally anchored rating scales. *Anecdotal notes* are written data about employee performance. *Open-ended essays* are written descriptions of employee performance. *Checklists* identify desired behaviors or activities, and rating scales assess each behavior on a numerical rating, usually from 1 to 5. *Behaviorally anchored rating scales* require the documentation of behaviors as well as a numerical ranking.

Commonly, evaluators err in evaluation. The most common evaluator errors are the halo effect, the recency effect, problem distortion, the sunflower effect, the central tendency effect, the rater temperament effect, and the guessing error. The halo effect occurs when evaluators' rank all categories high when an individual does well in several areas but not all. Recency effect occurs when the evaluator rates the employee based on recent events rather than the full year. Problem distortion is when the evaluator only remembers the problems with an employee's performance. The sunflower effect occurs when evaluators rate everyone high because they are part of a high-performance team, and central tendency effect is when the evaluator rates everyone average in order to avoid conflict. Rater temperament effect is when the boss errs on the side of leniency or strictness in evaluation, and guessing errors occur when the evaluator is behind in his or her work and estimates performance instead of collecting objective data.

Effective performance appraisal systems incorporate and enhance employee knowledge, skills, and abilities. Counseling is often used in cases where performance is substandard and work is poorly completed. Coaching is often used with employees to improve performance and learn new tasks or skills. Coaching can be role modeling, providing praise and information, or attendance at a seminar to learn new skills. Mentoring is also useful for employees who shine and demonstrate strong commitment and productivity.

LEARNING TOOLS

Activity

Purpose: To practice writing peer evaluations to include specific measurable data.

Scenario: Hillary is a hard-working RN who consistently provides excellent quality care to her assigned clients. She always helps others when her work is completed and has good working relationships with physicians, families, and other health care workers. One area Hillary despises is charting. She charts in a cursory, objective style, but does not always document everything that is needed. Rarely does she contribute to the nursing care plan, which necessitates others completing this work. Hillary is active in the Oncology Nursing Society and regularly attends continuing educational offerings. She has joined the unit-based quality improvement committee and contributes valuable information.

Directions: Below you will find a form that you must complete as Hillary's peer evaluator. Remember to make the notations as objective as possible. Descriptions of each category are listed below the client behavior and Likert scale. A Likert scale is used to rank her performance with a range of 1 for outstanding to 5 for unsatisfactory.

When making comments about Hillary's performance, use specific measurable objective data. For example, a comment in the professional development section might read: Hillary has been a member of the unit-based quality improvement committee for four months and attends regularly. Hillary has brought many ideas for improving processes on the unit, such as walking rounds instead of report, flexible hours for employees, and the need to develop procedures for new oncological treatments.

Clinical Behaviors

Client Care 1 2 3 4 5

Refers to client care activities such as personal care, treatments, medication administration, and coordination of care with physicians and other health care workers.

Comments:

Teamwork 1 2 3 4 5

Works with peers, physicians, clients, and other health care workers to maximize positive client outcomes and improve quality.

Comments:

Client Teaching 1 2 3 4 5

Individualizes a teaching plan for each assigned client, documents the teaching, and reports teaching needs during shift report.

Comments:

Committee Participation 1 2 3 4 5

Actively participates in at least one unit-based committee. Contributes to the committee process by chairing a committee, providing information for committee work, or completing the work of the committee.

Comments:

Charting 1 2 3 4 5

Documents timely, accurately, and comprehensively all client care activities, medications, and treatments.

Comments:

Nursing Care Plans 1 2 3 4 5

Initiates care plans for newly admitted clients during the shift of admission, updates, and modifies nursing care plans.

Comments:

Professional Involvement 1 2 3 4 5

Dresses professionally, participates in professional organization activities, attends continuing educational seminars, and provides leadership in unit-based activities.

Comments:

CASE STUDY

Stephanie is a nurse manager of a 75-bed oncology unit in large teaching hospital in Atlanta, Georgia. Stephanie has been a nurse manager at this hospital for 15 years and has developed a high-performance team on her unit. She personally interviews all applicants for her unit and encourages staff participation in the final selection. Stephanie frequently volunteers for pilot projects and is able to garner resources for staff projects. Stephanie finds performance evaluations difficult and has decided to rank everyone the same this year because they all perform so well as a team. She has decided to rank everyone high.

Case Study Questions

1. What type of evaluator error has Stephanie committed?
2. What are some other methods of evaluation that could assist Stephanie to make choices about employee ranking?
3. How could Stephanie use the performance appraisal process to assist the staff to individualize their learning needs as well as to meet organizational objectives?

LEARNING RESOURCES

Discussion Questions

1. What is the purpose of annual performance appraisals, and how should a nurse manager go about collecting objective data?
2. Is objectivity possible in a performance appraisal system? If so, how can a nurse manager make the appraisal process as objective as possible?
3. What are the current trends in annual performance appraisals in regard to who has what kind of input into employee evaluations?
4. In your organization, are employee performance appraisal ratings tied to monetary rewards? Or are the performance appraisal ratings used for self-improvement, and an across-the-board raise is given to employees? Which system of reward would motivate you?
5. Do you feel comfortable in providing and receiving peer evaluation? Do you find peer evaluation useful in upgrading your skills?

Study Questions

Matching: Write the letter of the correct response in front of each term.

_____ 1. Performance appraisal
_____ 2. Peer review
_____ 3. Absolute standard
_____ 4. Comparative standard
_____ 5. Anecdotal notes
_____ 6. Open-ended essays
_____ 7. Checklists
_____ 8. Rating scales
_____ 9. Behaviorally anchored rating scales
_____ 10. Sunflower effect
_____ 11. Performance
_____ 12. Performance management
_____ 13. Counseling
_____ 14. Coaching

A. Evaluations reference-based with other employee performance
B. List of desired employee behaviors
C. Rating everyone high because they are part of a high-performing team
D. Ratings based on documentation of employee behaviors
E. Evaluation based on the manager's own values
F. Paragraph descriptions of employee behaviors and performance
G. Numerical scores for assessing employee behaviors
H. Written records of employee behaviors
I. Evaluating the work of others
J. Assessing the level of work by an associate
K. Addresses problem performance such as substandard work
L. Is used to improve employee performance and their ability to do their job
M. Achieving or surpassing organizational and social objectives and responsibilities
N. An interactive process among work motivation, performance appraisal, and performance rewards and development

REFERENCES

Hersey, P., Blanchard, K.H. & Johnson, D.E. (1996). *Management of organizational behavior: Utilizing human resources* (7th ed.). Upper Saddle River, NJ: Prentice-Hall.

Nauright, L. (1987). Toward a comprehensive personnel system: Performance appraisal—Part IV. *Nursing Management, 28(2)*, 29-32.

SUPPLEMENTAL READINGS

Anderson, P. & Pulich, M. (1998). Making performance appraisals work more effectively. *Health Care Supervisor, 16(4)*, 20-27.

Campbell, D.J., Campbell, K.M. & Chia, H. (1998). *Merit pay, performance appraisal, and individual motivation: An analysis and alternative, 37(2)*, 131-46.

Kurtz, S.C. (1998). Human resources. Performance appraisal in the new health care environment. *Surgical Services Management, 4(9)*, 51-52, 54.

Martin, D.C. & Bartol, K.M. (1998). Performance appraisal: Maintaining system effectiveness. *Public Personnel Management, 27(2)*, 223-230.

Timmreck, T.C. (1998). Developing successful performance appraisals through choosing appropriate words to effectively describe work. *Health Care Management Review, 23(3)*, 48-57.

ANSWERS TO TEXT STUDY QUESTIONS

Chapter 17—Performance Appraisal (p. 343)

1. **What experiences have you had in the past with performance appraisals? Have those experiences been positive or negative? Why?**

   You may have had experiences with performance appraisals either as an employee or as a manager. Recipients of performance appraisals that have been positive cite being given the opportunity to discuss personal, professional, or organizational factors that either interfered with or augmented performance. Collaborative goal-setting with the manager results in a motivational process for employee growth and performance enhancement. In addition, positive recipient experiences with performance appraisals may serve as a template for conducting one's own future employee performance appraisals.

2. **Why does the handling of the performance process leave an aftermath of feelings?**

   A performance appraisal is an evaluative process that is very personal. You are being evaluated on your level of performance. The evaluation process used to quantify your performance may be influenced by perceptions, biases, and values of both the employee and manager. As a result, the opinions of the evaluator and yourself may differ. This difference in opinion may be a source of fear and anxiety because the appraisal may not truly reflect your perception of your performance. If the evaluation is positive, you will probably feel rewarded and motivated to continue a high level of excellence.

3. **Think about those times when you were evaluated in a positive and constructive manner. Why was that a good experience?**

   Performance appraisals that have been positive and constructive are those that provide an opportunity for personal evaluation, peer assessment, and collaborative goal-setting. The most important component in this type of evaluation process is the ability to conduct a self-assessment. A personal evaluation allows the individual to critically examine one's accomplishments and to identify areas for further growth. The collaborative goal-setting process with the manager can assist the individual to identify and implement strategies for professional development.

4. **How do you feel when you are expected to evaluate others? Why?**

   Evaluating others is a learned skill that requires time and experience to develop. Objectivity is essential, with the focus of the evaluation on counseling, performance improvement, and mutual goal-setting. Developing the employee's motivation to excel, stimulating professional growth, and enhancing skill mastery is an ongoing process that requires mentorship and continuous feedback.

5. **How are performance appraisal and quality improvement related?**

   Performance appraisals and quality improvement share many of the same process steps, including data collection, standards comparison, needs assessment, and mutual goal-setting. Both processes are concerned with outcomes management and the monitoring of actions that affect the quality of care.

6. **How should pay, promotions, and other rewards be tied to performance and its evaluation?**

   Salaries, promotions, and other rewards should be tied to the individual's performance and should be based on outcomes. Knowledge, skill, professional development, and the individual's accomplishment of goals should serve as the basis for the reward. Data should be collected, quantified, and documented throughout the evaluation period for objective presentation by the evaluator.

7. **How do you evaluate the performance of a team?**

   Although effective team evaluation may be problematic, it is possible. A team evaluation should be based on team strengths, accomplishments, and demonstration of team motivation and cohesion. Instead, the tendency is to evaluate individual performance of the team members; however, this does not appraise how those individuals worked together and solved problems as a team.

Collective Bargaining

STUDY FOCUS

In business and commerce, two groups, management and labor, often interact to resolve conflicts and negotiation over the terms and conditions of employment. Federal and state laws, administrative agency regulation, and judicial decisions regulate collective bargaining. The National Labor Relations Act (NLRA) enacted in 1935, signed by Franklin Roosevelt, is the main body of law for collective bargaining in the United States. The NLRA covers most private nonagricultural employees for the selection of a union for those who wish to engage in collective bargaining. This same legislation prohibits employers from interfering with the employee's selection of a labor union. The National Labor Relations Board was created from the NLRA with the two main functions of conducting representative elections and certifying results and preventing employers and unions from engaging in unfair labor practices. The Federal Service Labor-Management Relations Act (FSLMRA) governs federal employees and the Railway Labor Act covers the railway and airline industries for collective bargaining activities.

Areas of concern with nursing's involvement in collective bargaining includes the question of the appropriateness of nurses engaging in collective bargaining, the differences in the public and private sector arenas, and the NLRB and U.S. Supreme Court's decisions affecting nurses' inclusion in collective bargaining. Definitions that are important in the collective bargaining process are numerous. *Arbitration (interest)* is the use of an impartial third party to seek a solution to a dispute between parties involving the content of the collective bargaining agreement. The decision by the arbitrator is usually binding on the parties involved. *Arbitration (grievance)* is the use of an impartial third party to settle a dispute between the parties as to the meaning and application of certain language in the collective bargaining agreement. The decision of the arbitrator is usually biding on both parties. *Bargaining agent/representative* is the organization that the employees in a bargaining unit select to represent the employees in that unit in negotiations with the employer. Frequently there is a local bargaining unit that is affiliated with a national group. *Bargaining unit* is the group of employees who are joined together by the authorized agency to bargain collectively with the employer. *Certification* is the official designation by the labor agency of a bargaining agent as the exclusive representative of employees concerning matters of employment with management. *Collective bargaining* is the process used by representatives of an employer and the certified bargaining agent to write and sign an agreement covering terms of employment. *Contract* is the written agreement between the employees in a bargaining unit and the employer regarding the conditions of employment. *Good faith bargaining* is the performance of the mutual obligation of the employer and representative of the employees to meet at reasonable times and confer in good faith to conditions of employment. *Grievance* is the allegation by an employee or certified bargaining agent that management has violated the collective bargaining agreement. *Grievance procedure* is a written plan outlining the actions to be taken by both employees and their certified bargaining agent and the employer in order to adjust a grievance. *Impasse* is a deadlock in negotiations between management and employee representation over the terms of employment. *Management rights* are policies or practices that the applicable laws indicate are not subject to negotiation. *Mandatory bargaining items* are policies or practices that the applicable laws indicate management must negotiate with employee representatives.

Mediation is the use of a neutral third party to facilitate negotiations between employees and the employer. *Nonmandatory bargaining items* are policies or practices that applicable law indicates management may negotiate with its employees' agent. *Prohibited bargaining items* are policies or practices that the applicable law indicates management may not negotiate with its employee's agent. *Unfair labor practice* is an allegation made by an individual, an employer, or a labor organization of a violation of the law pertaining to collective bargaining.

In 1947 the Taft-Hartley Act amendments maintained the exclusion of not-for-profit hospitals, but in 1974 further amendments to the Taft-Hartley Act removed this exemption. There continues to be the issue of professionalism versus unionization for the profession of nursing. The American Nurses Association promotes economic and general welfare for nurses through the state nurses' associations representation of nurses as their labor union. More often than not, nurses unionize because of job satisfaction issues in an oppressive hospital environment. Unionization offers protection of workers, a unified voice, and opportunities to grow professionally.

Nurses must determine who will represent them in collective bargaining as well as who will be included in the bargaining unit. The NLRB clearly identifies those activities from which the employer must refrain from and the rules that labor unions must keep. The NLRB also describes the scope of bargaining that employees and employers must honor. Collective bargaining units are mechanisms to limit employers' capability of making unilateral actions. Nurses have joined unions to enhance job security as major health care reorganizations, layoffs, and downsizing have become the norm. In the 1990s, the U.S. Supreme Court ruled that nurses who supervise lower level personnel were supervisors and were therefore not protected by federal laws on collective bargaining under the NLRA. In 1996, the NLRB ruled that registered nurses including charge nurses were not supervisors and therefore were permitted to engage in collective bargaining. A concern that nurses still have is the lack of protection of their employment if they choose to be "whistleblowers." When nurses question the quality of care when staffing is consistently short or when the staffing mix is not adequate for the acuity level, they may risk losing their jobs.

LEARNING TOOLS

Group Activity

Purpose: To become knowledgeable regarding the collective bargaining activities within health care organizations that affect nursing practice.

Directions: Contact your state nurses' association and request information about collective bargaining activities within your state. Review the materials that the state nurses association distributes. Have each member of the group interview a nurse that they know about the issue "professionalism versus unionization" and the major issues they face in their day-to-day work. Write down the benefits and the limitations that nurses verbalize about unionization. If the nurses do not support unionization ask them what strategies or mechanisms they will use in the health care setting that they work to resolve conflict and negotiate desirable employment conditions.

Professionalism Versus Unionization Worksheet

Benefits of Unionization	***Limitations of Unionization***
______________________	______________________
______________________	______________________
______________________	______________________
______________________	______________________
______________________	______________________
______________________	______________________

Issues Faced in the Health Care Setting

____

____

____

____

____

____

____

Strategies to Resolve Conflict and Enhance Employment Conditions

Review the information that each group member collects and separate into two groups to debate the pro's and con's of professionalism versus unionization. Use the responses from the nurses who were interviewed to support each position.

CASE STUDY

Suzie is an exceptional registered nurse on the neurology unit at Billings Hospital in Montana. She is often charge nurse and consistently is able to answer all patient related questions and assist coworkers throughout the day. Whenever Suzie is in charge the work flow on the neurology unit is smooth and staff enjoy their work. Suzie works 7-3 shift, but is well respected on all shifts and on all units in the hospital. The nurses at Billings Hospital have become dissatisfied with the lack of recognition and control in what they consider to be an oppressive hospital environment. Wages have been kept low, unlicensed assistive personnel have been replacing registered nurse vacancies, and acuity levels are high on most units. Administration representatives seem to be ignoring the nurses' concerns. Suzie has been approached by several of the registered nurses at the hospital about organizing informational meetings with collective bargaining representatives. Suzie's coworkers would like her to take the leadership initiative for unionization at the hospital.

Case Study Questions

1. What should Suzie do? Should she take the leadership initiative and assist with informational meetings?
2. What are the issues that the nurses face? Are there alternative solutions to unionization? If so, what are the alternative solutions?
3. What are the advantages and disadvantages of unionization?

LEARNING RESOURCES

Discussion Questions

1. What are the tensions between the views of collective bargaining and its relationship to professionalism?
2. Discuss the history of collective bargaining as it pertains to the profession of nursing.
3. What are the major legislative acts that define collective bargaining?
4. What is the role of the American Nurses Association in collective bargaining?
5. What are factors that may influence nurses to engage in collective bargaining activities?

Study Questions

Matching: Write the letter of the correct response in front of each term.

_____ 1. Collective bargaining
_____ 2. Grievance
_____ 3. Mediation
_____ 4. 1974 amendments to the Taft-Hartley Act
_____ 5. National labor relations act
_____ 6. Bargaining unit
_____ 7. Contract
_____ 8. Impasse
_____ 9. Arbitration
_____ 10. Certification

A. A deadlock in negotiations between management and employee representation over the terms of employment
B. The official designation by the labor agency of a bargaining agent as the exclusive representative of employees concerning matters of employment with management
C. The use of an impartial third party to settle a dispute between the parties as to the meaning and application of certain language in the collective bargaining agreement
D. The main body of law for collective bargaining
E. The allegation by an employee or certified bargaining agent that management has violated the collective bargaining agreement
F. The use of a neutral third party to facilitate negotiations between employees and the employer
G. The process which is used by representatives of an employer and the certified bargaining agent to write and sign an agreement covering terms of employment
H. The removal of the exclusion of not-for-profit hospitals to engage in collective bargaining
I. Group of employees joined together by the authorized agency to bargain collectively with the employer
J. The written agreement between the employees in a bargaining unit and the employer regarding the conditions of employment

SUPPLEMENTAL READINGS

Breda, K.L. (1997). Professional nurses in unions: Working together pays off. *Journal of Professional Nursing, 13(2)*, 99-109.

Crippen, D.M. (1999). Medical economics and professional unions. *Cost & Quality Quarterly Journal, 5(1)*, 21-22.

Ketter, J. (1996). Issues update: Collective bargaining comes of age. *American Journal of Nursing, 96(12)*, 62-63.

McCullough, C. (1995). Collective bargaining: Empowerment and change. *Journal of the New York State Nurses, 26(1)*, 44-45.

ANSWERS TO TEXT STUDY QUESTIONS

Chapter 18—Collective Bargaining (pp. 354–355)

1. **Is it unprofessional to join a labor union? Why or why not?**

   There is controversy within the nursing profession regarding the congruency between professionalism and unionization. Some argue that unionization diminishes the nursing profession, equating unions to forums for less educated, blue-collar employees. Management intimidation, management allegiances, and union militancy contributed to the perspective of unionization as nonprofessional. However, others contend that collective bargaining serves to protect nurses and clients, while enhancing nurse professionalism, especially when conflict resolution, group solidarity, and collaborative decision making are used as strategies. An important consideration for nurses is the selection of an appropriate bargaining agent that can address their professional needs. Nurses may select union representation by a professional organization such as the American Nurses Association or one of its state organizations, or a traditional labor union such as the AFL-CIO. The choice of a bargaining agent that is knowledgeable about professional nursing practice and standards of care provides a better position to address the special interests of nurses than using industrial labor unions.

2. **Should not-for-profit hospitals be excluded from collective bargaining?**

   Legally, public hospitals are not exempt from collective bargaining. Collective bargaining involves negotiations between management and a group of employees, represented by a bargaining agent. An organizational culture that supports professional nursing practice, encourages participatory decision making, and creates a positive work environment may minimize the need for collective representation.

3. **Should nurses be allowed to strike? Why or why not?**

   A strike is a strategy used when the negotiations between management and the collective bargaining representatives reach an impasse that goes unresolved for an extended period. The decision to implement a strike is often an ethical dilemma for nurses. Typically, when the decision to strike is made, it has to do with more than economic compensation. Most nursing strikes are implemented because nurses believe that client safety and care delivery is being threatened. While a strike is not the best strategy for conflict resolution, sometimes it may be the only one that will enable nurses to maintain control over nursing practice and ensure the delivery of safe, quality health care.

4. **Does going out on strike amount to abandonment of clients?**

   Even though a strike is a problematical situation, it does not mean that nurses have abandoned their clients. When the decision to initiate a strike has been made, a walkout does not begin immediately. The collective bargaining representatives are required to give a 10-day written notice of intent to strike so that the health care organization may plan accordingly. In addition to implementing strategies to avert a strike, management begins to decrease client census, elective admissions, and routine surgeries. Scheduling plans are developed to cover certain units such as critical care, emergency, and surgery with nonunion nursing personnel.

5. **What other options besides unionizing are available for labor-management conflict resolution?**

   Besides unionization, labor-management conflicts can be resolved through effective human resource management and shared governance models. Open communication and employee empowerment in an organizational culture that values its staff will promote a positive work climate, quality client outcomes, and job satisfaction. The frequency of labor-management conflicts will be reduced in an organization that has satisfied employees who participate in the decision-making process.

Critical Thinking Skills

STUDY FOCUS

The health care environment is turbulent, constantly changing and chaotic. Nurses, as knowledge workers, encounter environmental stressors that require critical thinking skills for high-quality decision making. Nurses go through five stages of competence: novice, advanced beginner, competent, proficient, and expert. Critical thinking is reasoning that generates and examines questions and problems. Critical thinking is central in making sound clinical judgments. The development of critical thinking dates back to Socrates, who developed a questioning approach to thinking more clearly with greater logical consistency. Great thinkers like Plato, Aristotle, Thomas Aquinas, Francis Bacon, and Descartes also emphasized the need for critical thinking where individuals used a systematic disciplining of the mind to guide thinking.

Critical thinking requires logic, breadth, depth, accuracy, and relevance. Critical thinking questions include Why? What can I infer from this data? What is the most fundamental issue? Characteristics of critical thinking are disciplined, self-directed, accurate, and intellectual. The two cognitive processes used in critical thinking for nursing judgments are analytical and intuitive (Polge, 1995). Eight elements of purposeful critical thinking include clearly stated problem, goal identified, clear point of view, assumptions evident, concepts and principles used, data is collected, interpretations and lines of reasoning lead to conclusions, and implications and consequences result (Kelley, 1999).

Traditional thinkers tend to maintain the status quo, whereas critical thinkers challenge and question the norm. Traditional thinkers use problem solving, whereas critical thinkers ask *why* and challenge the "routine." Traditional thinkers choose solutions that are comfortable and familiar. Critical thinkers seek alternative solutions and take risks in choosing possible solutions. Critical thinking is associated with creative thinking. Creative thinking is the formation of novel ideas, products, or services. Three attributes of creative thinking are knowledge is received a whole, awareness of knowledge is immediate, and knowledge is acquired independent of linear reasoning (Benner & Tanner, 1987; Polge 1995). *Creative problem solving* is oriented toward achieving goals in novel ways (LeStorti et al., 1999). Creative problem solving is based on the principles of deferred judgment and divergent-convergent thinking sequence. *Deferred judgment* refers to the temporary suspension of criticism or evaluation of an idea. *Divergent-convergent thinking sequences* are an opening up of potential possibilities with the selection of the best option.

A *problem* is a deficit or surplus of something that is needed to achieve one's goals. We encounter problems daily in our personal and professional lives. Some situations produce problems (a difficulty), some problems create conflict (a dilemma), and sometimes an individual's solution does not take a logical path (a paradox). Solving problems effectively is important to making good client care decisions. Solving problems is a rational-logical thought process. There are six steps in the problem-solving process. The first step is to gather information from a variety of sources and to analyze that data. The second step is to define the problem by clarifying the task and describing it in a single sentence. The third step is to develop potential solutions in order to make the best choice. The fourth step is to consider the consequences for each of the identified potential solutions. Making the best decision is the fifth step. Finally, implement the solution, evaluate its effectiveness, and take necessary corrective action.

The *Kirton Adaptation-Innovation Theory* identifies two types of problem-solving styles, adapting and innovating. Adaptors use more traditional approaches to problem solving. They do not seek out problems to solve, but do resolve the problems they confront. In contrast, innovators seek novel situations, challenge rules, and create solutions. They discover problems and attack them vigorously. Problem solvers typically assess problems by their urgency and their immediacy. Some people envision problems on a time continuum. On one end of the continuum is a potential problem, which may emerge at any time; in the middle are actual problems that require prompt attention; and on the far end are critical problems, which are extremely urgent and require crisis intervention.

There are many strategies that can be used to solve problems. Some of the most common problem-solving strategies include direct intervention, indirect intervention, delegation, purposeful inaction, and consultation or collaboration. Direct intervention involves you personally doing a task or activity. Indirect intervention requires good interpersonal skills such as negotiation, conflict resolution, persuasion, and confrontations to influence others to carry out activities or resolve the problem. Delegation is used to assign the responsibility of an activity or task to another for the purpose of workload distribution. Purposeful inaction is consciously ignoring or choosing not to make a choice with the hope that the problem may go away with time. Inaction can be useful in some situations. Consultation or collaboration is exchanging information with peers and colleagues in order to solve a problem.

In today's health care environment, team-based approaches to patient care are commonplace. Nurses must learn to function and solve problems effectively in group environments. Dailey (1990) describes a nine-step problem-solving procedure to solve problems in group/team settings. The steps include: 1) identifying problems, 2) determining perceptions, 3) determining the underlying causes of problems, 4) assessing the magnitude of the problem, 5) constructing a plan, 6) implementing a plan, 7) test piloting the plan after discussing it with the team, 8) tracking effectiveness by creating indicators, and 9) publicizing results.

LEARNING TOOLS

Self-Assessment: Problem-Solving In-Basket Exercise

Introduction: Nurses are confronted daily with multiple problems, not only in their personal lives, but in their professional work as well. Diagnostic reasoning and clinical decision making are skills needed by all registered nurses. In-basket exercises are useful for improving skills.

1. Read the memos below, and then identify which problem type they are—potential, actual, or critical.
2. Take the critical problem you identify, and use the six-step problem-solving process to work it through. This exercise will give you practice in identifying types of problems and skill in solving them.

   You arrive on the unit, check your mail, and find the following memos:

Memo 1

From: Nancy, head nurse, 4 West

To: Sue, staff nurse

Re: Quality Improvement

Sue, as the 4 West representative to the hospital's quality improvement team, one of your responsibilities is to monitor documentation on the nursing flow chart, and alert and assist nurses to comply with our unit standards. In the most recent report, I noticed that 4 West has a poor rate of compliance. Please attend to this situation immediately.

(What type of problem is this? actual **)**

Memo 2

From: Jon, personnel director

To: Sue, staff nurse, 4 West

Re: Health Insurance

Sue, it has come to my attention that two of your health insurance enrollment forms were incorrectly completed. We have submitted the required data, and you have insurance coverage, but the records should be completed properly sometime in the future.

(What type of problem is this? potential **)**

Verbal Report 3

Sylvia stops you in the hall and tells you that Mrs. N.'s family is displeased with her care. They are demanding to speak to someone in charge. Sylvia is in a hurry to get home because she has a sick child and quickly leaves.

(What type of problem is this? critical **)**

Directions: Determine the most critical of the three problems identified above. Write the name of the problem below. Then use the six-step problem-solving process to resolve it.

Problem-Solving Steps

Decision Name:

1. Gather information.

Pt. left incontinent - situation assessed - Ask family + pt. + nurse.

2. Define problem.

3. Develop solutions.

Offer bedpan ac+pc, call bell, bedside commode,

4. Consider consequences.

Pt. dependency on staff, Skin breakdown, pt. + family satisfaction solutions won't work.

5. Make a decision.

Implement all 3 solutions.

6. Implement and evaluate solution.

Pt. skin is clean, dry + intact.

CASE STUDY

Beth is a nurse manager for the cardiac intensive care unit in a large teaching hospital in Birmingham, Alabama. She enjoys challenges, pushes her staff to maximum productivity, and works at least ten-hour shifts. If the organizational rules are in her way, she challenges them and works toward an innovative solution to the problem. Beth enjoys novel situations rather than routine or day-to-day challenges. She seems to thrive on unique problems and designs creative solutions to solve them. The staff on the cardiac intensive care unit like Beth's style and support her in her efforts.

Case Study Questions

1. According to Kirton's Adaptation-Innovation Theory, what type of problem-solving style is Beth exhibiting?
2. Describe the similarities and differences of adaptors and innovators.

LEARNING RESOURCES

Discussion Questions

1. What is the association between critical thinking and creative problem solving and how can these strategies be used in solving health care problems?
2. In what situations would a nurse use the problem-solving process as opposed to the team problem-solving process?
3. How do the steps of the problem-solving process, the nursing process, and the team problem-solving process differ? How are they similar?
4. What are some strategies that can be used to solve problems? Give examples of a situation in which these strategies would be useful.
5. Is it important for nurses to have diagnostic reasoning and clinical decision-making skills? If yes, why?
6. Should nurses consider the economic implications when providing client care?

STUDY QUESTIONS

Matching: Write the letter of the correct response in front of each term.

_____ 1. Problem solving
_____ 2. Actual problem
_____ 3. Adaptor
_____ 4. Innovator
_____ 5. Delegation
_____ 6. Potential problem
_____ 7. Critical problem
_____ 8. Critical thinking
_____ 9. Creative problem solving

A. A situation that is highly urgent and needs crisis intervention
B. A situation that is tenuous and difficulties can occur at any time
C. A situation that occurs in real time and needs prompt action
D. Assigning responsibilities and tasks to others
E. Uses tried and accepted solutions to problems
F. Uses innovative, creative solutions to problems
G. Using a process to identify obstacles and to achieve goals
H. Reasoning that generates and examines questions and problems
I. A novel approach to thinking to accomplish a goal

True or False: Circle the correct answer.

T F 1. Problem solving is a rational-logical thought process.

T F 2. It is inappropriate for a manager to use indirect intervention to solve problems.

T F 3. Purposeful inaction is an extremely valuable tool in most situations.

T F 4. Creative thinking is described by knowledge is received as a whole, awareness of knowledge is immediate, and knowledge is acquired independent of linear reasoning.

T F 5. A critical thinker preserves the norm or status quo.

REFERENCES

Benner, P., & Tanner, C. (1987). Clinical judgment: How expert nurses use intuition. *American Journal of Nursing, 87(1)*, 23-31.

Kelley, T.A. (1999). Critical thinking for case managers. *Inside Case Management, 6(5)*, 10-12.

LeStorti, A.J., Cullen, P.A., Hanzlik, E.M., Michiels, J.M., Piano, L.A., Ryan, P.L. & Johnson, W. (1999). Creative thinking in nursing eduction: Preparing for tomorrow's challenges. *Nursing Outlook, 47(2)*, 62-66.

Polge, J. (1995). Critical thinking: The use of intuition in making clinical nursing judgments. *Journal of the New York State Nurses Association, 26(2)*, 4-9.

SUPPLEMENTAL READINGS

Bailin, S., Case, R., Coombs, J.R., Daniels, L.B. (1999). Common misconceptions of critical thinking. *Curriculum Studies, 31(3)*, 269.

Kaasboll, J.J. (1998). Teaching critical thinking and problem defining skills. *Education and Information Technologies, 3(2)*, 101.

Kirton, M. (1989). Adaptors and innovators: Styles of creativity and problem solving. London: Routledge.

Marquis, B.L. & Huston, C.L. (Summer, 1994). Decisions, decisions, decisions. *Advance Practice Nurse*, Spring-Summer, 46-49.

Wade, G.H. (1999). Using the case method to develop critical thinking skills for the care of high-risk families. *Journal of Family Nursing, 5(1)*, 92.

ANSWERS TO TEXT STUDY QUESTIONS

Chapter 19—Critical Thinking Skills (p. 374)

1. **How can critical thinking and problem solving be used in nursing practice?**

   Critical thinking and problem solving are cognitive skills used every day in nursing practice in a variety of situations and settings. For example, they can be used to assess the situation, determine the problem, plan the course of action, and evaluate the outcome. These intellectual processes guide the nurse in determining the complexity, urgency, and focus of the problem and in developing alternative and creative solutions.

2. **Identify a problem you are dealing with now. What is your feeling about this problem? How do you approach it psychologically?**

   How one feels about a problem is influenced by their education, experience, perspective, and socialization. Moreover, the approach selected to solve a problem may be influenced by one's personality-related problem-solving style that influences how one acquires, stores, retrieves, and transforms information (Kirton, 1989). The Kirton Adaptation-Innovation Theory (1989) identified two types of problem solving styles: adaptors and innovators. Adaptors seek solutions to a problem using conventional approaches, while innovators create novel and different approaches to problem solving. Innovators question current practices and promote change.

3. **Do you tend to respond to a problem emotionally or logically?**

   Since emotional responses to a problem may be rooted in fear, anger, or resentment, they may not adhere to a sound or rational process. However, logical responses do follow a rational approach to problem solving that include gathering information, defining the problem, developing solutions, considering the consequences, making a decision, and implementing and evaluating the solutions. Understanding one's problem solving style increases self-awareness, knowledge, and the opportunity for incorporating alternative approaches to one's problem solving repertoire.

4. **What strategy do you tend to use for problem solving? Are there other strategies to try?**

   Individuals tend to use strategies that have been successful in the past. No matter what your particular strategy, some alternatives to consider are direct intervention, indirect intervention, delegation, purposeful inaction, consultation, and collaboration. Direct intervention involves direct, personal involvement, whereas indirect intervention involves only circuitous involvement. Similarly, delegation involves allocating certain responsibilities to others, while purposeful inaction is the conscious, deliberate decision to not act. Lastly, consultation or collaboration problem solving strategies involve the active participation of peers and colleagues to creatively identify solutions and to solve problems.

5. **How does problem solving relate to leadership?**

   Nursing leaders incorporate problem solving skills and strategies to propose changes, motivate others, modify the work environment, and to challenge the status quo. Proficiency in critical thinking enables nursing leaders to ask pertinent questions, discern relevant from nonrelevant information, analyze options, and to develop and enact realistic and practical solutions to problems. Decisions are made that affect not only the organizational culture and climate, but also the work environment, nursing practice, and client care. Innovations require effective problem solving skills to garner the needed resources and support to enact change.

6. **How does problem solving relate to management?**

   Nurse managers use problem solving strategies to make decisions regarding the work environment. Managerial decisions related to leadership style, resource allocation, shared governance, and budgetary concerns require adept problem solving skills and expertise. The development and enhancement of problem solving skills is a critical component to the enactment of the nurse manager role.

Decision Making Skills

STUDY FOCUS

Influential leaders make effective decisions that optimize organizational productivity, resources, and market share. A decision is selecting among competing alternative solutions. *Decision making* is behaviors exhibited in selecting from among competing alternative solutions and then implementing activities to accomplish your goal. Decision making not only deals with problems, but opportunities, challenges, and leadership initiatives as well. Decision making has five core elements: identifying a problem, establishing criteria to evaluate potential solutions, searching for alternative solutions, evaluating alternatives, and selecting the best choice. Individuals frame problems in different ways. One way is to use a systems approach like those used in quality improvement processes where emphasis is placed on the organizational process and group problem solving. Another method of framing a problem is to view the decision as individual rather than organizational. In an individual problem, all responsibility, accountability, and decision-making authority rests with one person.

According to Wren (1974), there are ten steps in the decision-making process: 1) becoming aware of a situation, 2) investigating the nature of the situation, 3) determining the objectives of the solution, 4) determining alternative solutions, 5) weighing the consequences and relative efficiency of each solution, 6) evaluating various alternatives, 7) selecting the best alternative, 8) implementing the decision, 9) evaluating the solution, and 10) correcting the solution based on evaluation. Desired decisions can be categorized into the end point of either minimal or optimal. Minimal decisions use basic requirements and meet minimum standards. These decisions are often referred to as satisficing decisions as they satisfy basic requirements. Alternatively, optimizing decisions are carefully evaluated, competing alternatives are weighed, and the best choice is selected. Optimizing decisions often result in positive outcomes, patient and staff satisfaction, and enhanced financial stability for the organization. It is sometimes difficult for individuals to think creatively or step "out of the box" to design innovate solutions. These individuals fall into six common traps: anchoring, status-quo, sunk-cost, confirming-evidence, framing, and estimating and forecasting.

Nurses use the decision-making process for individual, clinical, and organizational problem solving. *Clinical decision making* or *clinical judgment* is decision making based on nurse and client interaction and goal setting. Some nurses use diagnostic reasoning in their practice. *Diagnostic reasoning* is a four-step process that includes attending to available cues, activating hypotheses, gathering data, and evaluating hypotheses with data until a diagnosis is reached (Elstein, Shulman & Sprafka, 1978). *Organizational decision making* is assessing and solving systems problems to attain agency goals. *Ethical decision making* is examining conflicts among ethical principles, resource allocation decisions, and values.

Administrative decision making is common under conditions of uncertainty; high risk; and allocation of human, financial, and/or material resources. Four types of administrative decision-making strategies include satisficing, incrementalism, mixed scanning, and optimizing. *Satisficing* is getting by, selecting a solution that is good enough. *Incrementalism* is a slow step-by-step approach to solving an immediate problem with progress toward an optimal course of action. *Mixed scanning* combines an opportunistic approach to problem solving with the goal of optimizing the results. *Optimizing* entails choosing the course of action with the highest payoff.

One may engage in many different strategies when making decisions. Formal decision strategies include trial and error, pilot projects, problem critique, creativity techniques, the decision tree, the fish bone or cause-and-effect chart, group decision making, cost-benefit analysis, and worst-case scenarios. Trial-and-error strategies involve selecting the first available solution and trying it on the problem. Many times this approach results in poor outcomes. Pilot projects are mini-representations of a formal project. One unit is selected to implement the project, thereby minimizing risk and providing an opportunity to identify problems. *Problem critique* is a technique where a decision maker describes a potential solution for the problem to a friend or colleague, and then they critique the solution. Multiple creativity techniques include nominal group, Delphi, and brainstorming. The goal of creativity techniques is to identify as many potential solutions as possible without threatening individuals or critiquing responses. A *decision tree* is a graphic model of a problem's options, outcomes, and risks. *Critical paths* are examples of decision trees. *Fish bone* or *cause-and-effect charts* are graphic figures, diagrammed as a sentence is, with horizontal and slanted lines. The diagram represents the product, process, and outcome. Fish bones are used to diagnose causes of production problems. *Group decision making* is a process that engages the group to take ownership for organizational problems. *Cost-benefit analysis* is the process of identifying the costs and benefits of a solution to determine the fiscal, human, and material impact. Driving and restraining forces are also identified. Worst-case scenarios are typically used when money or prestige is at stake. Decision makers examine all possible events that could go wrong in order to determine a course of action that will protect the organization.

Nurses may also use the tools of perception and innovation in their decision making. These tools enable nurses to break out of their traditional decision-making strategies by finding novel solutions that provide a high payoff. Perception affects how one views the solution. Reframing one's perception of the problem or solution can create a new method to solve problems and may lead to the creation of a new device or new business. Innovations are those activities that have not been tried before in the same form. Reframing problems and solutions is a key strategy to change the way we perceive and select solutions.

Leadership is needed in designing decision support tools enabled by automation to standardize customized performance measures and quality outcome data. Effective leaders will be able to manage the concerns about health care error and client safety issues in the U.S. health care system by evaluating systems and creating new methods to ensure the safe delivery of quality health care. Maloch (1999) identified seven steps to determine an optimal course of action. Individuals should clarify the situation, identify goals, select measures, identify options, consider trade-offs, select the most congruent option for the goals, and evaluate the choices.

LEARNING TOOLS

Group Activity: Understanding Decision Making

Purpose: To identify the different types of decisions and to determine which decision situations are more appropriate for individual and group decision making.

Directions: For the three decision situations described below, identify the type of decision (administrative, clinical, or ethical), and who the appropriate decision maker is (individual or group).

Decision 1

Mr. Smith is in a nursing home. He is 72 years old and had a cerebral vascular accident three months ago which left him comatose. Mr. Smith has a feeding tube, and tube feedings are given on a regular basis. Mrs. Smith visited today and stated that she does not want you to give him tube feedings anymore because he wouldn't want to live "like this." What should you do?

Type of Decision ethical

Decision Maker individual/group to the ethics committee.

Decision 2

Mr. Jones returned from surgery eight hours ago. He had a left total knee replacement and now is complaining of excruciating pain. He is requesting pain medication. What should you do?

Type of Decision clinical

Decision Maker individual.

Decision 3

You are the team leader on an orthopedic unit for the 3-11 shift. All the nurses have been complaining of being overworked. At 11:35 p.m., all the nurses are gathered at the exit waiting for you. They are upset and demand that something be done about the chronic short staffing. What should you do?

Type of Decision administrative

Decision Maker individual/group.

As a nurse, you will be confronted with the need to make many different decisions. Determining quickly which decisions you can act upon by yourself and determining which ones need to be handled by a group is crucial to your success.

CASE STUDY

Dawn is a nurse manager for the operating room of a small community hospital in Oshkosh, Wisconsin. Dawn is required to make many administrative decisions daily. Dawn prefers to make administrative decisions by using a step-by-step approach to solving immediate problems, using solutions that fit into her long-range goals. For example, staffing problems have arisen in the operating room. Dawn's long-range goal is to have a mix of technicians and registered nurses in the operating room to provide quality perioperative care. Today, Dawn will begin discussing her plans with the staff, but in the meantime, will cover the staffing need with an experienced registered nurse from intensive care to assist in covering the holding room area. Dawn's experience suggests that taking small steps to solve a problem is useful and allows time to reflect on opportunities and barriers.

Case Study Questions

1. In administrative decision making, there are four strategies commonly used to make decisions. Which is Dawn using?
2. Describe the other administrative decision-making strategies.
3. What style of decision making is Dawn using? What style is most effective for this situation?

LEARNING RESOURCES

Discussion Questions

1. How can you use the tools of perception and innovation in your nursing practice?
2. What is the difference between an individual and organizational problem? Give an example of each.
3. Describe the formal strategies of decision making, and provide an example of a situation in which each would be useful.
4. Discuss the problem-solving and decision-making processes. Are there similarities? Differences?
5. What types of decisions should clinical nurses make? To whom should a clinical nurse turn for assistance in decision making?

Study Questions

True or False: Circle the correct answer.

T F 1. Clinical decision making is the same thing as diagnostic reasoning.

T F 2. Organizational decision making focuses on system problems.

T F 3. Ethical decision making is influenced by each person's values.

T F 4. Administrative decision making focuses on clinical problems.

T F 5. Critical pathways are a form of a decision tree.

T F 6. Group decision making tends to be more effective for system problems.

T F 7. In most cases, satisficing leads to effective decision making.

T F 8. Administrative decisions tend to be clear-cut and easy to solve.

T F 9. Decision-making strategies are interchangeable and can be used effectively in any situation.

T F 10. Pilot projects are full-scale implementations of a solution.

REFERENCES

Elstein, A., Shulman, L. & Sprafka, S. (1978). *Medical problem-solving: An analysis of clinical reasoning*. Cambridge, MA: Harvard University Press.

Malloch, K. (1999). The performance measurement matrix: A framework to optimize decision making. *Journal of Nursing Care Quality, 13(3)*, 1-12.

Wren, G. (1974). *Modern health administration*. Athens, GA: University of Georgia Press.

SUPPLEMENTAL READINGS

Boblin-Cummings, S., Baumann, A., & Deber, R. (1999). Critical elements in the process of decision making: A nursing perspective. *Canadian Journal of Nursing Leadership, 12(1)*, 6-13.

Caruth, D.L. & Handlogten, G.D. (1999). 8 mistakes to avoid in decision-making. *Manage, 51(1)*, 19-21.

Jacobs, S. & Pelfrey, S. (1995). Decision support systems: Using computers to help manage. *Journal of Nursing Administration, 25(2)*, 46-51.

Janis, I. & Mann, L. (1977) *Decision Making: A Psychological Analysis of Conflict, Choice, and Commitment*. New York: Free Press.

ANSWERS TO TEXT STUDY QUESTIONS

Chapter 20—Decision Making Skills (p. 393)

1. **What is your typical or preferred decision style?**

   Decision styles may range from autocratic, in which the leader makes the decision without input from others, to participatory, in which group members actively contribute to the decision. The selection of a given decision style depends on the presenting problem and the individuals involved in the situation. An effective decision maker has an array of decision approaches on hand to optimize positive outcomes.

2. **How does clinical decision making differ from managerial decision making?**

   While both forms of decision making involve the collection and processing of information and the selection and evaluation of an action, the focus of the decision differs between clinical and managerial decision making. Clinical decision making focuses on client issues or problems and nursing interventions. The sophistication of clinical decision making differentiates the professional nurse from the technical nurse. Managerial decisions focus on the resolution of organizational problems or the achievement of organization goals. An example of a managerial decision is the containment of costs while maximizing health care delivery.

3. **How are problem solving and decision making related to nursing?**

   Nursing uses problem solving and decision making skills for client care outcomes. These cognitive skills are routinely incorporated into the practice of both clinical and managerial nurses. All nurses collect information, draw conclusions, derive a course of action, and evaluate outcomes. Clinical nurses use these cognitive strategies to select the best nursing intervention, while nurse managers incorporate them in organizational decisions. Problem solving and decision making strategies are integral to maximizing patient outcomes and achieving organizational goals.

4. **What important decisions do nurses make? On which ones do they collaborate?**

   Nurses make many important decisions relative to the provision of care and care management. For example, nurses devise an array of strategies to optimize patient recovery, mobility and self-care, maintain airway patency and hemodynamic stability, and prevent the development of decubitus ulcers. Nurses collaborate on complex client care issues that require the talents and perspectives of a variety of health care professionals in order to maximize client outcomes. More specifically, nurses collaborate with the colleagues from the disciplines including medicine, social work, pharmacy, and pastoral services to address complicated and difficult client care problems. Nurse managers collaborate with other disciplines to achieve organizational goals, implement multisystem change processes, and to improve service delivery and client outcomes.

5. **What strategies work best for clinical decision making? For managerial decision making?**

   Nine decision making strategies have been identified: trial and error, pilot projects, problem critique, creativity techniques, decision tree, fish bone or cause-and-effect charts, group problem solving and decision making, cost-benefit analysis, and worst-case scenario. Because trial and error is considered a poor and risky option, the adept problem solver rarely selects it. Pilot projects are limited experimental trials used to develop an optimal and alternative solution to a problem, whereas cost-benefit analysis involves listing the positive and negative aspects of a given outcome to assist with decision making. Critical pathways, decision trees, and algorithms are commonly used protocols that guide the nurse through the decision making process. They describe activities that must occur in order to achieve a desired and predictable outcome. However, a caveat to remember is that the decision rendered may only be as good as the critical pathway, decision tree, or algorithm from which it was derived. Nurse managers select the best strategy considering the individuals involved and the given situation. For example, fish bone or cause-and-effect charts may be an effective strategy for nurse managers to select in examining possible causes related to production, while cost-benefit analysis may be an appropriate strategy to enlist when deciding budgetary issues.

6. **How can information processing help nurse decision making?**

   Professional nursing practice applies nursing expertise and knowledge to solving problems and making decisions relative to client care and care management. Nurses make decisions based on data collection, classification, storage, retrieval, and analysis (information processing). Using this process, nurses can develop creative solutions to issues and problems related to client care. Quality decisions depend on the data collected at the beginning of the problem solving process. Therefore, it is imperative that nursing data be clearly identified, definitions and measures clearly described, and data sets be standardized and accessible to support fiscal and clinical decisions. Patient care outcomes depend on quality data.

7. **What resources are available to assist with ethical decision making?**

Several resources are available to assist nurses with ethical decision making. For example, the American Nurses Association has published several statements that address this issue: Code for Nurses (1985), Social Policy Statement (1995), and professional standards of practice. Similarly, the Midwest Nursing Research Society's Guidelines for Scientific Integrity (1996) can also be used to resolve ethically sensitive scientific issues. One's personal, professional, and organizational values may assist with ethical decision making. Additionally, input from spiritual and religious leaders, multidisciplinary ethics committees, ethical decision making models, and the ethical principles of autonomy, beneficence, fidelity, justice, nonmaleficence, and veracity are available to guide ethical decision making.

8. **What creative or innovative ideas do you have?**

Creative ideas are central to innovations in nursing and health care. Innovative nurses examine situations from novel and different perspectives and devise creative and proactive approaches to a problem or dilemma. Nursing is replete with ingenious and resourceful minds that have potential to be on the forefront of clinical and organization changes to propel us into the future as a strong and powerful profession. We all have a contribution to make. What is yours?

Financial Management

STUDY FOCUS

Health care services are costly and pressures to control spiraling costs are growing. The target of financial management is to allocate scarce resources efficiently and effectively. *Financial management* is a set of activities involving the allocation of resources to complete organizational objectives and ensure viability. Four phases of financial management are budgeting, recording, reporting, and evaluating. To maximize the use of limited resources, organizations engage in planning. Operational plans are those activities determined necessary for meeting day-to-day organizational goals. *Strategic planning* is more long term and entails analyzing and projecting future organizational goals. A budget puts planning into financial terms and provides direction for managers. A *budget* is a written plan of revenues and expenditures. *Expenses* are those costs incurred to meet organizational goals. *Revenues* are payments made by patients and insurance companies for services rendered or an amount still owed for a service that was provided. *Profits* occur when revenues exceed costs of labor, materials, and overhead expenses.

Financial management of any organization occurs in the context of the broader community. The key factors to assess in communities are the major employers, provider groups, and health care facilities in the area. A population-based approach to planning health care services is essential. Other factors important in financial management include the structure of the health care organization, economic principles, and accounting and finance. *Economics* is based on principles related to the finite and limited nature of resources coupled with competing needs. There are two types of accounting: managerial and financial. *Managerial accounting* is the generation and evaluation of financial information needed to manage the organization. *Financial accounting* is providing information to external sources for investments, money lending, or control. *Cost accounting* or *cost analysis* is measuring and reporting costs. A *unit of service* is the basic measure of the product or service being produced. Costs may be fixed where they do not change as the volume changes, variable where they vary directly with volume changes, or marginal where there is extra cost of one more unit of service.

The core of organizational financial efforts are in planning and controlling resources through strategic planning, budgeting, and control of operating results. The elements of health care finance include taxes, philanthropy, operating finances, and capital financing. Strategies to avoid further escalation of overall health care costs include cost containment, avoidance, and reduction strategies. Problems faced in health care organizations include cash shortages, overstaffing, poor use of present staff, low productivity, and equipment breakdown. Research has shown that the reliability of service is the most important factor in judging service quality. Organizations depend on credibility of the services to maintain customer loyalty and survive.

Cost-effectiveness analysis can be used as a tool to evaluate the cost impact of new models of care. Decentralization is one strategy to empower and to motivate employees to increase accountability and productivity. A *cost center* is the smallest functional unit that generates revenues and expenses. Administration is one cost center that does not generate revenues. A *charge* is the price asked for services provided. *Cost* is the actual amount of money to cover direct production of expenses associated with the provision of the service. A profit is the money earned in excess of the charges over costs for providing a service.

Nursing service costs in the 1980s were 25 to 35 percent of the total budget. Because of the large size of nursing services in health care organizations and the view that nursing services are costs rather than revenue streams, nursing services are often targeted when cuts are made. Nurses must design new approaches to capturing revenues and demonstrating nursing contributions. Although administration costs have been estimated at 22.9 to 34 percent of the total budget, they have not faced the same scrutiny as nursing when cost cuts are made.

The nurse manager's role in financial management includes determining resource requirements, justifying resources, evaluating technology, and holding down expenses. The staff nurse's role in financial management includes contributing data and rationale for resource needs, practicing cost awareness in nursing care delivery, and understanding the basic techniques of financial management.

In all organizations, there will be competing demands for scarce resources. Conflicts and ethical dilemmas over competing demands for finite resources will abound. Examples of scarce resources in organizations include money, personnel, space, and time. Ethical obligations of fidelity, an obligation to act in good faith, and uphold trust and confidence can create conflicts for the nurse with patient, physician, and organizational needs competing for the nurse's loyalty. Aspects of an ethical practice environment include autonomy, trust, and communication. Great service companies build a humane, ethical, and value-driven community.

LEARNING TOOLS

Activity

Purpose: To examine and use financial management principles in the initial stages of developing a nurse-based business.

Directions: Work as a group to determine the key components of financial management when initiating a business. After group members determine the "business" and "services" that will be the "core" of the organization, use financial management principles to determine if the services will be used in the community. Use a population-based assessment to determine community needs.

Use the four phases of financial management to assist in organizing and planning for your company's future. Determine for each service provided the actual cost of producing the service, the charge you will collect, and the profit that will be generated. Determine the likely volume and then multiply it by the charge to determine revenues. Deduct all expenses: personnel, materials, overhead, and uncollectible amounts for services to determine potential viability. Don't forget to include the amount of start-up costs that will be needed to cover the period of time before revenues are generated.

Once the group has worked through financial management of a new business venture, discuss the following questions:

1. What are the similarities and differences in costs for a new business versus an existing business?
2. How can strong financial management assist in maintaining the organization's viability?
3. What factors are important in financial management?
4. What are businesses that nurses could initiate and own that would be profitable and serve community needs?
5. What Web sites provide data that can assist with financial management?

CASE STUDY

Holly, a nurse director of inpatient and outpatient medical-surgical services and the emergency room in a large teaching hospital in Santa Fe, New Mexico, has reviewed financial documents and is aware of a potential deficit in revenues in the emergency room cost center. Factors contributing to the projected deficit are an increase in uncompensated visits in the emergency room, increased turnover of registered nurses, and a relatively flat payment schedule from third-party payers on nonurgent patient visits. The volume in the emergency room has increased for nonurgent visits by 12 percent. Uncompensated visits account for the majority of this increase. Holly must make recommendations to the vice president of nursing to prevent the emergency room costs from getting out of control. Holly identifies three potential options: (1) hire nurse practitioners to staff a "fast track" for nonurgent patients; (2) partner with a free-standing urgent care center to refer nonurgent patients to their facility; and (3) institute a cost-cutting program in the emergency room.

Case Study Questions

1. What is the problem in this case study?
2. What financial management strategies could Holly implement?
3. What are other options that Holly might consider implementing in the emergency room?
4. What strategies would be useful to motivate staff to assist in implementing a potential solution?
5. Should financial data be shared with emergency room staff to assist in understanding the situation?

LEARNING RESOURCES

Discussion Questions

1. What is the role of the nurse manager and staff nurse in financial management?
2. Are the terms *budgeting* and *financial management* interchangeable? Why or why not?
3. What are the phases of financial management? What is included in each phase of financial management?
4. What are the types of accounting? Provide a definition and example for each.
5. What are the core elements of organizational financial planning and control? Why is each of these elements important?
6. What are the elements of health care finance?
7. What are scarce resources in organizations?

Study Questions

Matching: Write the letter of the correct response in front of each term.

_____ 1. Profit
_____ 2. Cost
_____ 3. Charge
_____ 4. Financial accounting
_____ 5. Managerial accounting
_____ 6. Unit of service
_____ 7. Cost center
_____ 8. Cost effectiveness analysis
_____ 9. Strategic planning
_____ 10. Financial management

A. The smallest functional unit that generates revenues and expenses
B. The price asked for services or goods
C. The actual amount of money required as payment to cover direct production inputs used in producing the services
D. Money gained as excess of charges over outlay costs in producing a service
E. Focused on the generation and evaluation of financial information needed by managers to manage the organization
F. Targeted to provide information to external sources of investments, money lending, or control
G. Focused on cost measurement and reporting
H. The basic measure of the product or service being produced
I. A series of activities designed to allocate resources and plan for the efficient operation of an organization
J. Process of assessing the organization and its departments

SUPPLEMENTAL READINGS

Halley, M. & Little, A. (1999). Net one, net two: The primary care network income statement. *Healthcare Financial Management, 53(10)*, 61-63.

Hartley, L.A. (1998). Fiscally "fit" in a managed care system. *Nursing Management, 29(12)*, 23-27.

Hofmann, W. & Jones, W. (1999). Tough love: Ten questions to ask your CEO. *Trustee, 52(9)*, 27-28.

Kuotsai, T. (1999). Symposium on local economic development financing: Issues and findings. *Journal of Public Budgeting, Accounting & Financial Management, 11(3)*, 387-397.

ANSWERS TO TEXT STUDY QUESTIONS

Chapter 21—Financial Management (p. 406)

1. **How does financial management relate to leadership? To management and control?**

   Financial management is a series of activities designed to meet the economic needs of the organization. Visionary leadership is needed to incorporate financial data into a budget, to develop a strategic plan to manage scarce resources, and to control organizational costs.

2. **How much effort should nurses place on financial management activities?**

   The role of nurses in financial management has expanded over the years. As such, nurses play an integral role in the determination and justification of resources, the evaluation of technology, and the implementation of cost-containment strategies. Staff nurse awareness and effort into practicing judicious financial management will reduce monetary losses so that cost savings may be allocated to care delivery and service quality.

3. **What strategies can nurses use to influence financial decision making?**

   Nurses can use their clinical knowledge and expertise to influence financial decision making. As coordinators of care, nurses can minimize the duplication of services and reduce wasted health care resources. Nurses who are knowledgeable about the financial management process can use innovative strategies to design care delivery systems that enhance productivity, cost effectiveness, and customer satisfaction.

4. **How can nurses gauge the financial effectiveness of their practice?**

   Nurses can gauge the financial effectiveness of their practice by using measurable outcomes.

   As nurses begin to identify the cost of their services, the positive outcomes of their care, and the resultant cost savings, they will be able to demonstrate financial effectiveness.

5. **In what ways can nurses address legal or ethical issues arising in financial management?**

   Nurses can address legal or ethical issues associated with financial management by advocating for quality health care and patient safety, by upholding professional practice standards, and by following organizational policies and procedures. This process will be facilitated in organizations that foster autonomy, trust, and communication among its employees.

Outcomes Management

STUDY FOCUS

Florence Nightingale was the pioneer of systematic client outcomes evaluation through her collection and analysis of data on mortality for the improvement of health care in a hospital in Crimea. Today, it is imperative for nurses to collect data on outcomes measurement in order to provide evidence of effectiveness, efficiency, and cost benefits of services performed. The benefits of measuring health care outcomes include surviving in an unstable job market, improving the quality of care, informing health care consumers, and ensuring nursing's perspective is represented. Consumers are demanding to know the extent to which clients are benefiting from and satisfied with health care services provided.

Key terms in outcomes measurement and management include outcomes, indicators, outcomes measurement, and outcomes management. An *outcome* is the result of an effort to accomplish a goal. Outcomes are the end results of an effort. *Indicators* are valid and reliable measures. *Performance measures* are quantitative tools such as a ratio applied to a specific area in an organization's performance. *Outcomes measurement* is measuring the results of care. *Outcomes monitoring* is repeated quantification of data based on observation as opposed to measurement. *Outcomes management* is a multidisciplinary process to provide quality services, enhance outcomes, and constrain costs by using process activities to improve outcomes.

The goals of outcome management are to improve quality, reduce risks, decrease fragmentation, and constrain costs. The process of measuring outcomes is multifaceted and is initiated with the identification of the indicators of interest. Data are aggregated, analyzed, and interpreted. Changes are then implemented based on the outcomes and the process cycles with evaluation activities implemented. Factors influencing the demand for outcome measurement included the lack of existing outcome studies, the need for quantifiable health care data, and the variation among medical practices in the diagnosis and treatment of clients. In addition, employers were demanding to know not only the costs of health care, but what client outcomes were achieved for the dollars invested. Potential questions that outcomes data can answer in nursing include: What nursing interventions will achieve the best outcome for a specific symptom in a given patient population? What educational intervention is most effective in preparing clients for diagnostic interventions? What clinical pathway is most cost effective while maintaining high-quality care for the delivery of services for a specific population group?

Mortality and morbidity data were among the first outcomes that were measured. In the 1980s, the classic Medical Outcomes Study framework included end points, functional status, general well being, and satisfaction with care. The Joint Commission on Accreditation of Healthcare Organizations (JCAHO) developed the *Indicator Measurement System* to evaluate the quality of care provided by health care organizations. The Visiting Nurses Association developed the *Omaha System* that was originally intended to improve its client record system. The Omaha System incorporates a scale to measure knowledge, behavior, and status. The *Outcomes and Assessment Information Set* (OASIS) was developed to collect outcomes data in home care agencies. The National Committee for Quality Assurance developed the *Health Plan Employer Data and Information Set* (HEDIS). HEDIS was developed to provide a standardized system for managed care organizations to use in measuring and reporting quality performance.

Trends in outcomes measurement include the collection of complex, interactive, and multidimensional data across multiple levels. Multidisciplinary, cross-site investigations provide useful outcome data for improving the health and well being of communities. Leaders in health care must provide direction in outcome management to ensure detailed descriptions of important outcomes. Nurses must continue to analyze outcome data sensitive to nursing interventions, refine computerized data support for nursing-sensitive outcomes, and facilitate multidisciplinary teams toward comprehensive outcomes management.

Accurate and timely data are essential to effective leadership in outcomes measurement and management. Managers often evaluate the common cause of variability in order to manage services effectively. Tools to organize and visually display data to examine common causes of variation include Pareto charts, run charts, histograms, control charts, scatter diagrams, flow charts, and cause-and-effect diagrams. Outcomes measures for quality, service, and cost are important for employers, clients, and managers. Standardized report cards are being developed and used in health care organizations to improve quality, cost, access, and services. Standardized reports are also being used to compare health care organizations in communities.

LEARNING TOOLS

Assessment: Outcomes

Purpose: To analyze an organization's outcomes measures to determine if they are nursing sensitive.

Directions: Conduct a short interview with a registered nurse, charge nurse, and nurse manager on the unit to which you are assigned for clinical experiences. Ask each of the individuals the following questions:

Interview Format for Outcome Measures

1. What is the process used to collect outcome data for this unit? ______
2. How often is outcome data collected on this unit? ______
3. Who is responsible for collecting and analyzing the outcome data? ______
4. What are the outcome measures monitored for this unit? ______
5. How is the outcome data reported to the staff of the unit? ______
6. What interventions are implemented based on outcome data? ______

List the outcome indicators in two categories as to nursing sensitive or non-nursing sensitive.

Outcomes Measures by Category

Nursing-Sensitive Outcomes

______
______
______
______
______
______
______
______
______
______

Non-Nursing-Sensitive Outcomes

______
______
______
______
______
______
______
______
______
______

Add the total number of outcomes measures for the clinical unit. Are there more nursing-sensitive outcomes or non-nursing-sensitive outcomes? If there are more non-nursing-sensitive outcomes, what outcomes could be added to effectively measure nursing interventions?

Share the findings of the interviews with your colleagues. What did they discover? What are key outcomes for nursing?

CASE STUDY

Jill, a nurse manager for a mid-sized primary health care center in Carter, Wisconsin, conducted a clinical outcomes study on all clients diagnosed with diabetes, asthma, and hypertension. The outcomes measures were high for clients who had been diagnosed with hypertension and asthma. Clinical outcomes measures for clients with a diagnosis of diabetes were low. Jill was not surprised when the data showed that clients were meeting clinical outcomes when diagnosed with asthma or hypertension. Jon, a primary care physician, had developed a patient education system and managed most of the patients who were diagnosed with hypertension and Jen, a family nurse practitioner, had developed a patient education system and managed most of the patients who were diagnosed with asthma.

Case Study Questions

1. What is the problem in Jill's office?
2. Who should Jill involve when developing potential strategies to improve client outcomes of those with a diagnosis of diabetes?
3. Is process important in outcomes management? If so, how is process important?
4. What may be useful outcomes measures for those who have a diagnosis of diabetes?
5. How will clients, employers, and the providers in Jill's office benefit by improving the outcome scores for those who have a diagnosis of diabetes?

LEARNING RESOURCES

Discussion Questions

1. Should nurses collect indicators that are not sensitive to nursing? If so, why should they collect these indicators?
2. What is the proper balance between process and outcomes in the provision of health care services?
3. What outcomes measurement systems are there and what is the purpose of each of these systems?
4. What are the goals of outcomes management? How can outcomes management positively impact the profession of nursing?
5. What are nursing-sensitive indicators? Provide examples.

STUDY QUESTIONS

Matching: Write the letter of the correct response in front of each term.

_____ 1. Outcome
_____ 2. Indicators
_____ 3. Performance measures
_____ 4. Outcomes measurement
_____ 5. Outcome monitoring
_____ 6. Outcomes management

A. The result of care or end product
B. A valid and reliable measure
C. A quantitative tool
D. A multidisciplinary process that uses process activities for improving outcomes
E. Repeated quantification of outcomes data based on observation of indicators
F. Measuring the results of care

True or False: Circle the correct answer.

T F 1. The Health Plan Employer Data and Information Set was designed for outcomes measurement in home care agencies.

T F 2. Outcomes management provides relatively little data for internal use within health care organizations.

T F 3. The majority of outcome data collected in health care organizations is nursing sensitive.

T F 4. The lack of documentation of effectiveness of client services and the variations in practice have triggered the demand for outcomes measurement.

SUPPLEMENTAL READINGS

Hansten, R. & Washburn, M. (1999). Seven steps to shift from tasks to outcomes. *Nursing Management, 30(7)*, 24-27.

Kamrad-Marrone, S.L., Stabile, M.A. & Smeltzer, C.H. (1999). Understanding and championing the merger process: Key leadership roles for successful outcomes. *Nursing Administration Quarterly, 23(4)*, 47-57.

Pelletier, L.R. (1998). Outcomes management Internet resources. *Journal of Nursing Care Quality, 13(1)*, 1-7.

Randy, J. Lewis, K.A. & McCall, D. (1998). A multistakeholder-driven model for developing an outcome management system. *The Journal of Behavioral Health Services & Research, 25(2)*, 151-162.

ANSWERS TO TEXT STUDY QUESTIONS

Chapter 22—Outcomes Management (p. 417)

1. **Are outcomes more important than processes?**

   The outcomes of care provision have always been a focus for nurses. Although outcomes are an important measure of quality service and client care, delivery processes cannot be ignored or discounted. The path or mechanism used to achieve desired outcomes may reveal insightful or disturbing revelations regarding the attainment of outcome goals. By examining processes, modifications and adjustments can be made to the current system in order to make it more efficient, effective, and client-focused, while actualizing desired outcomes.

2. **Do outcomes equal quality?**

   Although related, outcomes and quality are two separate entities. Outcomes in health care are the result of providing care, whereas quality is a measurement of how well care was given. However, quality is a difficult phenomenon to measure because it holds different meaning for different groups. For example, clients, health care professionals, organizations, and regulatory agencies may view the concept of quality from a different perspective. Organizations and insurance companies may view quality from a resource management or cost effectiveness perspective, while clients and families may evaluate quality by degrees of satisfaction. Health care professionals may assess quality by the amount of time and staff available for the delivery of personalized care.

3. **What are the key indicators and outcomes for nursing?**

   Traditionally, morbidity and mortality rates were used to measure the outcome of nursing care. In addition to death and disease, other outcomes included assessment of disability, dissatisfaction, and discomfort. More recently, outcomes measures have expanded to include psychological, physiological, functional, behavioral, knowledge, home functioning, family strain, safety, symptom control, quality of life, goal attainment, client satisfaction, cost and resource allocation, and resolution of diagnosis. Examples of nursing quality indicators include incidence of patient injury, occurrence of nosocomial infections, presence of pressure ulcers, and the frequency of medication errors.

4. **Are outcomes measures defined consistently across organizations?**

   Several governmental and accrediting agencies have created outcome measures that are used across organizations. Databases have been developed to evaluate outcomes for Medicare and Medicaid recipients, the quality of care provided by large health care organizations, and the effectiveness of nursing care. In order to identify trends and initiate changes that will improve the quality of care delivered and reduce risk, it is imperative that outcome measures be compared by organizational location, size, and clientele. Differences in clients' health status and the presence of co-morbid conditions, as well as staffing ratios and personnel mix may explain variations in outcome measures between organizations.

5. **How do you know if an outcome is sensitive to nursing?**

   Efforts to develop outcomes that are sensitive to nursing were initiated in the past two decades. Nursing's initial efforts to quantify its contribution to the health care system included the development of standardized nomenclature necessary to obtain comparative nursing-sensitive data. A nursing-sensitive outcome is one that focuses on the care recipients and their perceptions, conditions, and behaviors that respond to nursing interventions.

6. **Should nurses ignore outcomes not sensitive to nursing?**

   Nursing must be cognizant of outcomes that affect the gamut of health care delivery. Moreover, nurses need to examine organizationally sensitive outcomes that may mask the positive impact of nursing care. As nurses make astute clinical decisions that maximize patient outcomes while reducing health care expenditures, the ability to discern the cost savings for the institution would provide data that were nursing sensitive.

Productivity and Costing Out Nursing

STUDY FOCUS

Productivity is key to organizational financial viability. Nurses are continually pressured to produce more with fewer resources. Research has shown that there are ten aspects that enhance productivity (Hernandez, et al., 1988; Janson, 1999). The aspects include participative decision making, open communication flow, concern for human resources, structure of the work group, increased peer leadership, supportive group processes, encouraging best efforts, increased preplanned activity, decreased information-processing requirements, and providing relevant services.

Productivity is the ratio of resources used to provide the service (input) to client outcomes or services (output). The administrative team in health care organizations is faced with decreasing reimbursement for services and with capitated payment systems. To compete effectively for market share, health care organizations must provide quality services at reasonable costs. Capitated systems require that organizations provide a package of comprehensive services to clients for a fixed fee per head. If health care organizations are to survive, they must provide the services effectively and efficiently. *Effectiveness* is doing the right things correctly to achieve established outcomes. *Efficiency* is providing the necessary services quickly and inexpensively.

Nurse managers must be cognizant of productivity levels and the cost of nursing services in order to manage a health care organization effectively. The term *costing of nursing services* refers to the cost of services or interventions carried out by nurses. *Nursing productivity* is a combination of nursing care hours and the provision of nursing care services. To increase productivity, nurses can provide services with fewer nursing care hours or complete more interventions in a shorter time period. The challenge is to increase productivity, ensure quality, and empower employees to improve processes. Substituting equipment for labor, improving work methods, removing unproductive practices, and improving human resource management can increase employee productivity.

Nurse managers must possess refined skills in calculating productivity. Calculating hours per patient day (HPPD) is the oldest nursing productivity index and is imprecise. Other methods include dividing input by output, dividing cost by unit of output, dividing dollars by worked hours, dividing nursing hours worked by the number of hospital client days, and dividing the number of nursing staff by census of client days. When determining productivity, both decision making and tasks must be included in workload calculations. Standards of care, time and motion studies, and job descriptions provide a basis for developing tools to collect workload data.

The cost-effectiveness and cost-benefit models assist in determining productivity. The *cost-effectiveness model* examines different methods of obtaining desired outcomes. It examines different programs whose objectives vary in order to determine the most productive method of providing services. The *cost-benefit model* is resource-driven, while the cost-effectiveness model is goal-driven. Productivity measures are complex because measuring nursing care outcomes is controversial. Nursing care and outcomes are not standardized, and a best method for resource use in nursing interventions is not clearly delineated.

Costing out nursing services is important in order to facilitate nursing's input in public health decisions, health policy, and reimbursement decisions. Costing out nursing services provides data to facilitate comparative productivity measures within and between organizations. Specific costs then can be determined for each nursing intervention and nursing diagnosis, which in turn further establishes a mechanism for determining third-party reimbursement. Organizational survival will depend on shrewd management and leadership in controlling costs, in empowering employees to improve and streamline processes, and in procuring resources for promising innovations.

Activity based costing is an approach to service costing that is different from traditional methods and may be useful in managed care and capitated reimbursement systems. This costing approach reflects what it costs to provide services and why costs were incurred. The two steps to activity-based cost assignment include identifying activities that consume resources and assigning activities to cost categories. Assignment of costs for activities are based on actual time spent by activity.

The Medicare Cost Report may also be used as a resource for costing out nursing services in hospitals. Hospitals being reimbursed with Medicare funds are required to submit annual data on cost-to-charge ratios. Hospital bills can be unbundled and both a cost and price for nursing services may be established.

An important strategy for enhancing productivity is the investment in infrastructure for computerization. The use of technology and computerization for productivity improvement designed to enhance communication, provide rapid documentation, and end-of-shift reports saves considerable nursing time and increases accuracy, but tremendous initial capital expenditures are required.

LEARNING TOOLS

Productivity Assessment

Purpose: To practice calculating simple productivity measures, and to understand the importance of productivity in health care organizations.

Methods for Calculating Productivity

A. $\dfrac{\text{OUTPUT (dollars)}}{\text{INPUT (work hours)}} = \text{P (productivity)}$

Explanation: Input can include supplies, equipment, labor, and overhead expenses for the building. This simple calculation provides insight into the work hours per revenue generated ratio. A nurse manager examines several items when reviewing monthly budget reports. Is the unit over budget in supplies, equipment expenditures, or labor? Are client days high, low, or on budget? All these factors will impact the amount of profit generated by the unit. Work hours divided by dollars gives one quick picture of labor expense to revenue generated.

OR

B. $\dfrac{\text{TOTAL COST}}{\text{UNIT OF OUTPUT (client days)}} = \text{P (productivity)}$

Explanation: The cost of managing the care of clients is based on multiple factors. One factor is the volume of clients for which care is provided. Another is the dollar amount required to provide that care. Try the following set of calculations in order to assess Unit A's productivity. First you need to know that Unit A's fixed cost to operate annually is $300,000 with a variable cost per day of $100 for each of the 6,000 client days.

Calculate the cost of each client day by combining the fixed cost and the variable cost ($ per day x # of client days) to reach the total cost. Then using the formula, divide the total cost by the output (# of client days) to find the total cost per client day. (See the end of the section for answers.)

Step one:

Step two:

Step three:

OR

C. $\dfrac{\text{COST OF DIRECT CARE}}{\text{WORK HOURS}} = \text{P (productivity)}$

Explanation: A cost per direct care hour can be determined by taking the total budgeted cost for the department and dividing it by the total budgeted direct client care hours. The cost per direct care hour is important because it indicates the average cost of care for a client. The direct care hour cost is usually based on productive (worked) hours.

Try the following set of calculations in order to assess Unit B's productivity. First you need to know that the total budgeted cost for labor for the unit is $600,000, and the total number of direct client care hours are 43,680.

Divide the total budgeted cost for labor by direct client care hours to get the total direct care hour cost.

Step one:

OR

D. $\dfrac{\text{NURSING HOURS}}{\text{\# OF HOSPITAL CLIENT DAYS}} = \text{P (productivity)}$

OR

E. $$\frac{\text{NUMBER OF NURSING STAFF}}{\text{CENSUS}} = \text{P (productivity)}$$

Explanation: The number of hours worked divided by the number of hospital client days reflects the acuity level of clients. This can be compared to budgeted levels of nursing hours per hospital day; from these numbers, the overall productivity level can be assessed.

Another approach is dividing the number of staff by the census of client days. This provides an overall staff to client ratio, which typically stays relatively constant. Deviation from the typical staff/client ratio gives a manager an indication of increased or decreased staff productivity.

Answer to B

Step one:
6,000 (client days) x $100/day = $600,000

Step two:
$600,000 (variable cost) + $300,000 (fixed cost) = $900,000

Step three:

$$\frac{\$900{,}000 \text{ (total cost)}}{6{,}000 \text{ (client days)}} = \$150 \text{ per client day}$$

Answer to C

$$\frac{\$600{,}000 \text{ (labor costs)}}{43{,}680 \text{ (direct client care hours)}} = \$13.74 \text{ dollars per direct care hour}$$

CASE STUDY

Karen, a nurse manager of a 23-bed step-down unit in a medium-size hospital in El Paso, Texas, prides herself on the fact that her unit has the highest quality scores in the hospital. The clinical staff who work on the step-down unit consistently document all nursing interventions and pertinent client data, carry out procedures according to protocol, and go out of their way to facilitate the client's journey to health and wellness. Many physicians use the step-down unit as an example of excellence in client care. The only problem that Karen has is keeping the unit on budget and maintaining a high level of productivity. In comparison to the other units, the step-down unit has a low productivity level and a high budget.

Case Study Questions

1. Is the unit Karen manages efficient?
2. Is the unit Karen manages effective?
3. What would you do if you were the manager? Would you maintain status quo or try to improve productivity?

LEARNING RESOURCES

Discussion Questions

1. What type of activities could help leaders increase employee productivity? What type of activities could help managers increase employee productivity?
2. What is productivity? How do you measure productivity?
3. What are the different types of reimbursement systems in health care today?
4. What are some changes that could be made on your unit in order to improve productivity?
5. What is the cost-effectiveness model? What is the cost-benefit model? Give an example of a situation in which you would use each of these models.
6. What is activity based costing and in what clinical setting would it be used? Provide a rationale for your answer.

Study Questions

True or False: Circle the correct answer.

T F 1. Productivity is measured by calculating the cost of nursing care multiplied by the unit of output.

T F 2. Effectiveness is how fast or inexpensive a service is provided.

T F 3. Efficiency is doing the right things to improve quality.

T F 4. Costing out nursing services is the actual cost of providing services by nurses.

T F 5. Time and motion studies are no longer valuable in determining workload requirements.

T F 6. The cost-benefit model is goal-focused and examines different methods to achieve outcomes.

T F 7. The cost-effectiveness model is a budgetary model that determines costs and assists managers with determining the proper skill mix for a unit.

T F 8. Economies of scale refer to the productivity of units.

T F 9. At the present time, doctors are reimbursed for services provided by nurses.

T F 10. Nurses are in a prime position in the changing health care environment and need only to sit and wait for expanded roles in managed care environments.

T F 11. The use of technology and computerization improves productivity and increases accuracy.

T F 12. Activity based costing is a useful approach to employ in the hospital setting.

REFERENCES

Hernandez, S., Kaluzny, A., Parker, B., Chae, Y. & Brewington, J. (1988). Enhancing nursing productivity: A social psychological perspective. *Public Health Nursing, 5(1)*, 52-63.

Janson, C.L. (1999). *Understanding organizational culture and increasing productivity {On-line}*. Available: http://www.nadona.org/understanding%20organization.htm

SUPPLEMENTAL READINGS

Cleland, V. (1990). *The Economics of Nursing*. Norwalk, CT: Appleton & Lange.

DeMoro, R.A. (1998). Medical stripmining and the new nursing shortage. *Revolution: The Journal of Nursing Empowerment, 8(1)*, 40-41.

Harris, R.M. (1998). Advanced nursing practice in the 21st century: Do we want to be right or do we want to win? *Online Journal of Issues in Nursing*. Available http://www.nursingworld.org/ojin/tpc6/tpc6_2.htm.

Price, D.M. (1998). An ethical perspective. Doesn't everyone want an efficient nurse? *Journal of Nursing, 5(1)*, 51-55.

Sengin, K. & Dreisbach, A. (1995). Managing with precision: A budgetary decision support model. *The Journal of Nursing Administration, 25(2)*, 33-44.

ANSWERS TO TEXT STUDY QUESTIONS

Chapter 23—Productivity and Costing Out Nursing (p. 430)

1. **Why would quality of care suffer when nursing care hours are reduced?**

   The quality of care services is influenced by a number of factors including the staff mix, the care delivery system, acuity levels, and the number of caregivers assigned to provide direct and indirect care. When nursing care hours are reduced, there is less time to perform all of the required client care activities. As a result, nurses are required to work faster, streamline documentation, or decrease client-centered activities. When nursing care hours are drastically reduced, the nurse may have to prioritize client care, completing the most urgent care first and leaving many client care needs unmet.

2. **Do more experienced nurses work more productively? Why or why not?**

   Productivity is based on many factors including knowledge, experience, motivation, administrative support, and commitment to quality care. Experienced nurses are generally more productive than novice nurses because they have more experience and a stronger knowledge base to make astute clinical judgments. If experienced nurses are not motivated, lack administrative support, or have serious personal problems, their productivity level may decline. As novice nurses gain experience, efficiency, and confidence in their clinical decisions, their productivity level increases.

3. **Why should nurses worry about productivity?**

   Nurses comprise the largest expenditure for health care organizations. When cost-cutting strategies are implemented, areas with large expenditures are targeted for reductions. If nurses are unable to demonstrate that they are productive members of the health care team and that they positively impact client outcomes, they will be targeted for workforce reductions.

4. **What issues in productivity are most urgent? Why?**

   It is important for nurses to standardize the measurement of productivity. Productivity measures are complex because quantifying nursing care outcomes is difficult, there are no clear relationships between care process and nursing outcomes, and the most efficient resources for performing care are unknown. Without standardization of productivity indices, meaningful comparisons among nursing units and facilities are not possible.

5. **How do nurses determine if their care is effective and efficient?**

   Effectiveness is doing the right things and achieving quality outcomes, whereas efficiency is how fast a service or product is completed in the most cost-effective manner. Nurses have established quality improvement programs that monitor indicators of care for compliance. Quality programs determine how effective the care has been. Efficiency is usually monitored by productivity measures. Costs are tracked by examining actual expenditures compared to budgeted projections, with adjustments for units of service or patient days.

6. **Why should nurses cost out their services?**

   Costing out nursing services is important so that nurses know the actual costs of services to clients. This knowledge is used for reimbursement decisions and to facilitate health policy formation. In order to obtain third-party reimbursement, nurses must be able to cost out nursing care, clearly articulate the outcomes of care delivery, and negotiate services for a set fee. Through these processes, nurses will be able to demonstrate their effectiveness and worth to the organization.

7. **How can nurses control health care costs? Nursing costs?**

   Several strategies can be used to contain costs. Effective leaders can motivate and collaborate with employees to find innovative methods to be productive, effective, and efficient in accomplishing the organization's goals. According to Sibson (1976), employee productivity can be increased by substituting equipment for human labor, improving work efforts, minimizing unproductive work practices, and improving human resource management. Case management of high-risk populations can control health care expenditures. Other health care costs can be controlled by providing community-based care and by using advanced practice nurses in primary care settings. Evaluating skill mix and care delivery systems, facilitating interdisciplinary collaboration, maximizing reimbursement, and using critical pathways to reduce redundancy can control nursing costs.

8. **What is the ideal ratio of nurses to clients?**

   Unfortunately there is no ideal ratio of nurses to clients. Nurse to client ratios are dependent on the acuity level of the patients, the education and experience of the nurses, the technology required for care provision, the work methods, the care delivery system, and information technology. Evaluating standards of care, conducting time and motion studies, and assessing client care requirements provide a foundation to determining the ratio of nurses to clients.

Organizational Climate and Culture

STUDY FOCUS

Examining an organization's culture and function improves nurses' effectiveness by providing useful information about the interpersonal and political forces in the organization that influences productivity and work operations. Assessing organizational culture is an important aspect of a nurse's role. Gaining an appreciation of cultural influences will improve a nurse's effectiveness by providing information about the interpersonal and political work environment. There are four viewpoints used when thinking about organizations — structural, human resource, political, and symbolic. A structural viewpoint focuses on the structure, roles, and relationships in organizations. The human resource perspective emphasizes the role, function, and integration of employees in the organization. A political view focuses on the allocation and distribution of constrained resources. In a symbolic view, those items that are not explained rationally are examined and meaning is attached to the situation.

Each organization has rituals, traditions, values, rules, and a structural component. Those shared beliefs, values, and practices that exist in an organization are organizational culture. Those perceptions that individuals hold about the environment are the organizational climate. Organizational culture is a more complex phenomena. It often is subtle and is not controlled by management. Management may influence culture by providing rewards and penalties, but a group to control its environment and to ensure safety and survival forms a distinct culture. Organizational culture serves four major functions. The first is to provide a sense of identity for group members. Secondly, it promotes a sense of commitment to the group. The third function is to enhance the stability of the group environment. Finally, it helps the group to make behavior understandable.

Several elements comprise the culture of organizations, including stories, myths, rituals, and ceremonies, as well as metaphors and analogies. These elements provide concrete examples, guidance, and communication for a culture. Stories often describe heroes or conflicts. Myths are rich descriptions of events that provide inspiration and enhance belief. Rituals are embedded customs that socialize new members, provide clear messages to members, and stabilize the culture. Ceremonies entail pomp and circumstance and are functions that benefit members and the group. Metaphors and analogies are used to explain complex phenomena by simplifying the explanation using information the member knows.

The three levels of culture are the visible level, which includes physical space and social surroundings, the values of the culture, and the basic underlying assumptions that guide behavior. Five critical elements of culture in an organization include the mission statement, formal structure, informal structure, political structure, and financial structure. Each of these five elements is critical in understanding how an organization functions.

Culture can be implicit or explicit. An explicit culture is more formal with rules, policies, and procedures clearly written and communicated. Norms and values are established. Implicit culture, on the other hand, is subtle and difficult to identify. Knowledge is not verbally shared, there are informal work rules, and people do not openly communicate their values and traditions. How then, can a nurse identify the culture on a unit? A cultural checklist is a beneficial tool to analyze organizational culture. The checklist should include the following: image, deportment, status symbol and reward systems, subcultures, environment and ambiance, communication, meetings, rites, rituals, and ceremonies, and sacred cows. Assessing organizational culture is an important first step in understanding how the organization functions. Once an analysis is completed, a nurse may choose to change or build the culture to incorporate positive values and beliefs. The strategies for building culture emphasize a basic framework of support. The first step is to start building from wherever the group is currently and to work from there. Establish personal contact, use all communication channels, and facilitate open dialogue and discussion with the group. Identify shared values and goals so the focus and desired outcome are clear. Jointly determine strategies and take action.

Positive work group cultures are important for nurse satisfaction and retention. Clinical nurses can work together to build networks and support systems for enhancing positive work environments and tackling thorny issues. Building positive cultures increases productivity and morale while improving quality client care. Effective leaders strategically influence organizational culture to enhance client-centered care and partnerships in a healthy work environment.

LEARNING TOOLS

Group Activity: Organizational Culture Analysis

Purpose: To examine the unit where you wish to practice when you complete your educational requirements. Use the following Organizational Culture Checklist to analyze the organization (the checklist has been adapted from the Huber text and is based on the elements described by del Bueno & Freund, 1986).

ORGANIZATIONAL CULTURE CHECKLIST

Aspects of Culture	Questions for Assessment
1. Image	How do the nurses dress? Casually or formally? What symbols or slogans are used? Is the unit aesthetically pleasing?
2. Deportment	What is the level of courtesy shown to clients' families? Are males and females treated equally? Are all health care workers treated with respect?
3. Status Symbols	Are the nurses' parking and lounges comparable to physicians' and administrators'? Is there an elitist attitude? If so, by whom? Are offices and equipment comparable?
4. Subcultures	Do nurses from the same cultural background tend to form friendships with each other more easily? Are there cliques on the unit? Are new employees welcomed by the group?
5. Environment and Ambiance	How well is the physical structure maintained? Is the decor attractive and well kept? Is there space for classrooms and lounges? Are rooms reserved for special groups?
6. Communication	How does the CEO communicate to staff nurses? Does the vice president of nursing make rounds on all units? How does the nurse manager share information with employees? Does the important communication take place in formal meetings or informally in groups?
7. Meetings	Who participates in which meetings? How are participants for meetings selected? How are decisions made in committee? Where are meetings held? Are refreshment provided?
8. Rites, Rituals, and Ceremonies	How are holidays celebrated? Is longevity recognized? What events are celebrated and recognized? What are the policies for orientation and termination?
9. Sacred Cows	Who are the heroes/heroines? What subjects are taboo? Are there policies that are untouchable?

The information you gather from your cultural assessment will provide you with a basic understanding of the organization's culture. You will be able to tell if the culture is explicit or implicit. You will be able to tell whether the organization is formal or informal, how policies and procedures are made, and the nature of interpersonal interactions among staff. This data will provide you with information useful in determining the type of unit where you wish to work.

CASE STUDY

Susan is a registered nurse on a 58-bed neurosurgical unit for a large community hospital in Portland, Oregon. She is working on a project concerning organizational cultural assessments as part of the requirements for her master's degree in nursing. Susan has discovered tension among the staff about their new roles after an organizational redesign. There is much resistance on the part of the staff members about "letting go" of their old responsibilities and taking new ones. Susan carefully examines the written communications including memos, policies, procedures, and job descriptions. She notices that many of the documents have not changed since the organizational redesign. Traditionally, the hospital has relied heavily on written documents to provide stability and guidance for the staff. Now, staff are feeling insecure and reluctant to change. What should Susan do?

Case Study Questions

1. Has the organizational culture where Susan works been explicit or implicit?
2. What organizational viewpoint is most evident in this culture?
3. What strategies should Susan take to realign the organizational culture?
4. What critical cultural elements must Susan examine?

LEARNING RESOURCES

Discussion Questions

1. To do an in-depth cultural assessment of an organization, how long would it take, and what criteria would you use to evaluate the organization?
2. What strategies could a nurse employ to change or build organizational culture?
3. What is the nurse's role in building organizational culture?
4. What is the difference between implicit and explicit culture? Which type of culture is easier to analyze?
5. What are the critical cultural elements in an organization, and how do they strengthen the existing organizational culture?
6. What is the nurse manager's role in influencing the unit culture? What strategies may be useful in producing the desired cultural change?

Study Questions

Multiple Choice: Circle the correct response.

1. Susan, an RN on the neurosurgical unit, is assessing organizational manifestations by cultural level. When she assesses the visible level, what is Susan examining?

   A. balance of cost, quality, and access to care

   B. physical space and social environment

   C. guidelines of the organization

   D. values of what ought to be in the organization

2. After Susan examines the cultural levels, she begins examining the five critical cultural elements in the organization. What five elements does she examine?

   A. values, mission statement, basic assumptions, and formal and informal structure

   B. mission statement; basic assumptions; and formal, informal, and political structures

   C. values; basic assumptions; and formal, informal, and political structures

   D. mission statement; and formal, informal, political, and financial structures

3. Susan knows that an organization needs a framework of support for building a culture. Which of the following are necessary components for supporting a culture?

   A. values, communication, actions, and strategies

   B. communication, values, strategies, and mission statement

   C. actions, strategies, mission statement, and shared values

   D. mission statement, strategies, actions, and communication

4. Susan decides to take a structural view of the organization in her cultural analysis. What data should she collect?

   A. data on the allocation and distribution of scarce resources

   B. existing symbols and signs in the organization

   C. the communication and interpersonal network in the organization

   D. the formal roles, relationships, and organizational structures

5. Susan is teaching a continuing education class on

organizational culture. Which of the following definitions should she use to define organizational culture?

A. shared beliefs, values, and assumptions that exist in an organization

B. perceptions that individuals have about the environment in the organization

C. gives meaning and significance to activities in organizations

D. every organization's values, rituals, and rules

True or False: Circle the correct answer.

T F 1. Climate may be called the organization's "personality."

T F 2. Examining an organizational culture improves nurses' effectiveness by increasing understanding of the interpersonal and political forces at work in the organization.

T F 3. As a shift in health care delivery occurs from acute care to community-based care the number and variety of jobs for nurses has decreased.

T F 4. Culture is a form of external group control and is based on beliefs about organizational survival.

T F 5. Culture enhances the stability of the social system.

REFERENCE

del Bueno, D. & Freund, C. (1986). *Power and Politics in Nursing: A Casebook.* Owings Mills, MD: National Health Publishing.

SUPPLEMENTAL READINGS

Coccia, C. (1998). Avoiding a "Toxic Organization." *Nursing Management, 29(5)*, 32-33.

Gilmartin, M.J. (1999). Creativity: The fuel of innovation. *Nursing Administration Quarterly, 23(2)*, 1-8.

Hemingway, M.A. & Smith, C.S. (1999). Organizational climate and occupational stressors as predictors of withdrawal behaviours and injuries in nurses. *Journal of Occupational and Organizational Psychology, 72(3)*, 285-299.

Hendry, J. (1999). Cultural theory and contemporary management organization. *Human Relations, 52(5)*, 557-577.

Shoou-Yih, D. & Alexander, J.A. (1999). Consequences of organizational change in U.S. Hospitals. *Medical Care Research and Review, 56(3)*, 227.

ANSWERS TO TEXT STUDY QUESTIONS

Chapter 24—Organizational Climate and Culture (p. 450)

1. **What is the relationship between an organization and its values?**

   The values of a given organization are a reflection of its culture and climate. Organizational values shape normative behaviors, perceptions, and social mores within the employment environment.

2. **To what extent does an organization's culture determine job satisfaction?**

   Organizational culture influences one's perception of the interpersonal milieu and working environment. Job satisfaction is related to the work environment. Personal congruence with the culture of the organization will positively affect job satisfaction; conversely, incongruence with the organizational culture will negatively affect job satisfaction.

3. **How can you assess an organization's culture?**

   Several mechanisms are available to assess an organization's culture. One can examine the traditions, rituals, ceremonies, myths, and rules that are present within the institution. The physical and social environments of the organization, the values, and the underlying assumptions of acceptable organizational behavior can be evaluated. Lastly, one can examine the mission statement, formal structure, informal structure, political structure, and financial structure, constituting critical elements of an organization's culture.

4. **How long does it take to really perceive the culture?**

   To examine and understand the many facets of an organization's culture is a time-intensive process. As such, it is difficult to quantify the exact amount of effort, observation, and interaction necessary to really understand the cultural milieu of an organization. One's own perspective, acceptance, and personal agenda may influence one's comprehension and evaluation of the organizational culture.

5. **Is caring the central value in nursing?**

   Caring has been identified as one of the central tenets of nursing and is often described as the essence of nursing. It is a core concept and considered the "normative glue" in nursing.

6. **What are the effects of leadership on culture?**

   Organizational leadership can shape, sustain, or change culture. Altering organizational culture can be an arduous and complex endeavor that requires mutual trust, respect, and commitment. Cultural change depends on four key elements: an awareness of current culture, an assessment of the current culture's conflict with the proposed change, a strategy to implement the change, and the use of incentives and rewards for supporting change.

7. **Does organizational culture reflect an individual's perception of the organization, or is it a relatively enduring characteristic?**

   Organizational culture develops over time and is resistant to change. Beliefs, values, and assumptions, the defining elements of a culture, are deeply embedded core convictions that require examination, reflection and thoughtful deliberation to amend. Cultural beliefs and values endure as long as they are accepted, supported, and perpetuated by group members.

8. **How can you build a culture?**

   Building a culture requires a framework of shared beliefs and values. To build a culture, one would start where the group currently is, establish open discussions, identify shared values and a mission, determine strategies, and take planned action.

9. **What is the best kind of organizational culture for nursing?**

   The best organizational culture for nursing is one that is respectful, supportive, and congruent with nursing's own beliefs, values, and assumptions. Organizational values similar to professional nursing values provide a work environment that provides a "good fit" for nurses. An example is the value of caring, which is reflected in the manner the organization treats its employees.

10. **What values are important in an entrepreneurial nursing environment?**

    Entrepreneurial activities are inspired in an environment that values trust, risk taking, open communication, access to information and resources, and employee worth. Organizations that support entrepreneurial activities encourage employee contribution, creative thinking, and innovation at all levels in the organization.

11. What nursing values create dilemmas?

Dilemmas are created when a conflict exists between individual values and beliefs and organizational expectations. This disparity causes internal conflict, despair, and discord. As a result, dilemmas arise that polarize organizational and personal expectations. Examples of issues that may precipitate a conflict between nursing and organizational values include staffing, costs, and client's rights.

Mission Statements, Policies, and Procedures

STUDY FOCUS

Organizations are composed of a group of individuals who each have specific responsibilities to act together toward the goals of the organization. Management to efficiently and effectively meet organizational goals and to provide direction to employees, vendors, and consumers provides organizational structure. Health care organizations are complex and require professional staff to accomplish their mission. The mission statement of the organization describes the product; for health care organizations the product is client care.

Organizations are social systems comprised of the environment and individuals. The environment is composed of the internal and external environments, roles, and goals or expectations. Individuals have their own needs, personalities, and personal agendas. At times, individuals' needs or desires may be in conflict with organizational goals. By accepting employment within an organization, employees imply that they will abide by the organizational philosophy.

Organizations have mission statements to guide the institution and provide direction to employees. *Mission statements* are composed of a philosophy, a purpose, and objectives. A *philosophy* is a statement of values and beliefs. It is abstract, describing a vision and providing guidance. The nursing department's philosophy should be congruent with the organizational philosophy and include the three vital components of client, nurse, and nursing practice. The purpose of the organization is its reason for existence. It spells out the service(s) to be provided. The nursing purpose must take into consideration the organization's purpose, the state Nurse Practice Act, and legal concerns. The objectives are hoped-for outcomes directing activities toward organizational goal accomplishment. *Objectives* must be behaviorally specific statements in written format. They must be realistic, attainable, and priority-focused.

Policies and procedures are written to clearly articulate the rules of the organization that are derived from the mission statement. Policies and procedures are developed to coordinate the work of the organization. *Policies* are general guidelines that speak to repetitive problems or tasks in the organization. The policies help coordinate plans, control performance, and increase the consistency of activities. Policies are usually written, although informal policies may exist. Policies speak to all employees and not just one job category. *Procedures* provide a step-by-step plan to complete a task. They are developed for those activities that recur on a regular basis, and they provide a performance guideline for them. Procedures are written, provide a reference, and are typically in a consistent format. The procedure format includes the purpose of the activity, the individual who is responsible for performing the activity, steps in the procedure, and supplies or equipment necessary to accomplish the task.

A positive work environment fostered by a philosophy that espouses group participation and commitment is paramount to a successful, effective team. A caring approach that focuses on common elements of successful organizations, that retains employees, and that includes a managerial commitment to employees, strong leadership, and competitive salaries and benefits fosters employee commitment. A value of caring and excellence for all constituents, clients, staff, and other health care workers enhances work commitment and quality outcomes. Support for autonomy, innovation, and risk taking is embedded in a team-building philosophy. In contrast, behaviors that create barriers to organizational excellence include telling versus asking people about their needs, depersonalizing members of the organization, acting without habitual courtesy, and showing contempt for individuals. These behaviors are exhibited by preferential treatment, insensitivity, a lack of communication, ambiguity in job requirements, and a user attitude toward employees.

LEARNING TOOLS

Role Play #1

Caring Behaviors that Build Teams and Promote Commitment

Character One = Jill is the vice president of nursing and frequently makes rounds on all 15 client care units in the hospital. Jill is supportive of all her staff and empowers them to make autonomous decisions. Clinical and administrative staff frequently consult with her on their projects.
Character Two = Jack is a clinical nurse who was hired three months previously and has been doing an outstanding job with clients, but he is having some problems interacting with residents.
Character Three = Joe is a resident and has just started working with one of Jack's clients. Joe has been at the hospital for one year and has been short with staff on occasions.
Character Four = Sally is a nurse's aide who is working with Jack to provide supportive care to the clients.

• • • • •

Jill is rounding on all the units when she hears voices beginning to rise. She turns the corner to see Joe, Sally, and Jack discussing a problem in loud voices.

Role Play Questions:

1. What should Jill do? Should she intervene? If so, what should she say?
2. What strategies could she employ using a caring approach to intervene?
3. How can she manage the situation to empower all of the individuals involved?

Role Play Worksheet

Characters	Student Assigned
Jill, the vice president of nursing	__________
Joe, the resident	__________
Sally, the nurse's aide	__________
Jack, the clinical nurse	__________

Which character have you been assigned?

What are your character's goals in this situation?

How can the other characters assist you in achieving your goals?

What might the other characters do to hinder you in achieving your goals?

What strategies and probes do you plan to use in this situation?

Role Play #2

Behaviors that Create Barriers to Organizational Excellence

Using the same characters (Jill, Joe, Jack, and Sally) and the same scenario (Jill rounds the corner to discover a problem), role play a situation using contempt behaviors that block effectiveness and increase turnover.

Role Play Questions:

1. What should Jill do? Should she intervene? If so, what should she say?
2. What strategies could she employ to create a barrier and disempower employees?
3. Discuss why individuals choose to use contempt behaviors to resolve problems.

Role Play Worksheet

Characters	Student Assigned
Jill, the vice president of nursing	________________
Joe, the resident	________________
Sally, the nurse's aide	________________
Jack, the clinical nurse	________________

Which character have you been assigned?

What are your character's goals in this situation?

How can the other characters assist you in achieving your goals?

What might the other characters do to hinder you in achieving your goals?

What strategies and probes do you plan to use in this situation?

CASE STUDY

Jacqueline is a newly hired vice president of nursing for a 250-bed hospital in Maine. She has carefully read the mission statement of the organization and decides to make rounds on the units to see how integrated it is on the units. The mission statement describes the hospital as a community-based center of excellence that provides care to all clients in a cost-effective manner. On her rounds, she stops to talk with Debbie and Karen, both of whom are nurse managers. She asks them what the mission of the organization is, and Debbie replies that it is to provide high-quality health care, and Karen says that it is to increase the market share for obstetrics patients. Jacqueline also asks several staff nurses about the mission statement and gets a variety of responses.

Case Study Questions

1. What purpose does a mission statement serve?
2. Is it a problem that nurse managers and clinical nurses are unable to recite or explain the mission statement?
3. What can Jacqueline do to increase employee awareness of the mission statement?

LEARNING RESOURCES

Discussion Questions

1. What are the differences between a philosophy, a purpose, and an objective?
2. How does the organizational philosophy relate to the nursing philosophy?

3. Are employees obliged to agree with or carry out the mission statement? If so, why?
4. How can nurse leaders promote positive work cultures?
5. What is the clinical nurse's role in developing philosophy, purpose, and objectives?

Study Questions

True or False: Circle the correct answer.

T F 1. An organization has a purpose, structure, and individuals.

T F 2. A philosophy describes the reason the organization exists.

T F 3. The purpose relates the values and beliefs of the organization.

T F 4. Objectives are outcomes that direct an activity toward goal accomplishment.

T F 5. The three core components of a nursing philosophy are the client, the nurse, and the physician.

T F 6. A policy is a step-by-step guide to solve common problems.

T F 7. A procedure is a general guideline that guides goal accomplishment.

T F 8. Caring philosophies empower individuals and assist in organizational goal attainment.

T F 9. Contempt behaviors create barriers to excellence in organizations.

T F 10. Nurses desire improvements in image, autonomy, and collaboration.

SUPPLEMENTAL READINGS

Graham, P., Constantini, S., Balik, B., Bedfore, B., Hooke, M., Papin, D., Quamme, M. & Rivard, R. (1987). Operationalizing a nursing philosophy. *Journal of Nursing Administration, 17(3)*, 14-18.

Nyberg, J. (1993). Teaching caring to the nurse administrator. *Journal of Nursing Administration, 23(1)*, 11-17.

Raven, J. & Rix, P. (1999). Managing the unmanageable: Risk assessment and risk management in contemporary professional practice. *Journal of Nursing Management, 7(4)*, 201-206.

Saner, R.J. (1999). Third-party biller compliance guidance emphasizes risk awareness. *Healthcare Financial Management, 53(3)*, 43-45.

ANSWERS TO TEXT STUDY QUESTIONS

Chapter 25—Mission Statements, Policies, and Procedures (p. 466)

1. **How do previous employee experiences color perception and attitude? Why do these perceptions linger?**

   The recency and vividness of the experience in conjunction with one's own values and beliefs affect how perceptions are derived and interpreted. Experiences with employees may be evoked when similar situations arise and used as the foundation for future decisions. These perceptions tend to linger as they are salient experiences that remain accessible in and retrievable from our memories.

2. **Do nurses profess loyalty to the organization/job or to the profession/work of nursing? Can an individual have both?**

   Nurses' loyalty to the profession of nursing germinates early in the formal educational process. Its values, beliefs, and traditions are internalized and incorporated into practice and leadership approaches. When nurses enter the institutional system, organizational loyalty is expected, requiring nurses to balance professional and organizational loyalties to find the most comfortable "fit." Similar values and beliefs support the ability of nurses to remain loyal to both their profession and their organization. However, conflicts in loyalty may arise if incongruent values and beliefs are present between the organization and the profession.

3. **How do you use the change process to implement a new philosophy in a preestablished work group?**

   Leadership involves establishing a philosophy that serves as the basis upon which innovative changes can be based, planned, and actualized. Understanding the readiness and willingness of a work group to adapt a new philosophy is key to developing strategies that will facilitate its successful implementation. Leaders can facilitate this process by motivating, guiding, inspiring, and supporting employees in the process of relinquishing old value and beliefs, and shaping a new philosophy.

4. **What is the "philosophy in action"? Cite some examples. Describe why this makes a difference.**

   Brown-Stewart (1987) described "philosophy in action" as subtle behaviors that demonstrate a lack of concern for people and an undermining of their success. Examples of such contempt behaviors include lack of habitual courtesy, withholding information, lack of education and orientation, and insufficient staffing. These behaviors decrease employee satisfaction, morale, and work performance, and negatively impact client outcomes and organizational accomplishments.

5. **What problems are solved by having policies and procedures?**

   Policies and procedures, extensions of the mission statement, are standards in the form of written rules that guide decision making and performance. As such, they provide structure, consistency, and stability so that nursing functions in a coordinated fashion, decreasing the amount of chaos present in the work environment.

6. **What decisions can nurses make without a written policy?**

   Some policies are unwritten, or implied, by patterns of decisions that have already been made within the organization. Professional nursing judgment is used when making client care decisions. However, when management or client care issues arise outside the scope of practice or expertise of the nurse, the nurse must contact the appropriate manager or professional colleague to assist with decision making.

Organizational Structure

STUDY FOCUS

The structure of the organization provides a framework for accomplishing the work of the organization. Organizational structure is essential for the efficient and effective management of work, power, and control in organizations. The structure of an organization is the way in which personnel are divided by their tasks and coordinated to accomplish organizational goals. Many factors are examined before organizational structures are designed. These factors include the age of an organization, its size, technology, internal and external environment, and its resources. There are both formal and informal organizational structures. *Formal structure* refers to what is clearly written into an organizational chart. *Informal structure* is the internal and external network of relationships and interdependencies around the organization. One aspect of the informal structure is the "grapevine."

Important concepts of management are associated with structure such as division of labor, span of control, scalar process, and line and staff positions. The *division of labor* refers to the assignment and distribution of the organization's work to individuals who have the authority and responsibility to complete the job. The *span of control* refers to the number of subordinates one manager oversees. The *scalar process* is the levels within the organization. *Line positions* are those in direct line of hierarchical authority and central to producing a product of the organization. On the other hand, *staff positions* provide the expertise and knowledge to meet organizational goals.

Mintzberg (1983) has identified technology, social environment, size, and task repetitiveness as major influences on structure. In health care, sophisticated technologies; rapid, complex decisions; and the changing professional workforce present a formidable challenge for administrators and require decentralized, autonomous teams working to promote quality client care. Organizational size changes as it ages. An organization begins with a small, organic, and unelaborate structure. The second stage is entrepreneurial directed by a dynamic, powerful executive. A formalized structure emerges, and a bureaucracy begins to form. As the organization ages and grows, divisional structures develop, and finally, it may shift to a matrix structure.

Health care organizations traditionally have used one of three basic types of administrative structures: bureaucracy, matrix, and adhocracy. Mintzberg (1983) addresses the basic coordinating mechanisms to accomplish work. They are mutual adjustment, direct supervision, standardization of work processes, standardization of work outputs, and standardization of worker skills. The more complex the environment, the more fluid and autonomous it is, needing little supervision.

Structures can be flat or tall. Tall structures are typically in a pyramid shape with the board of control at the top and the staff at the bottom. Board members typically control fiscal resources and make policy. Within each level of the pyramid, there are positions. The terms *position* and *job* are often used interchangeably; however, there is a difference between them. A job is composed of a collection of positions that encompass the same basic configuration of tasks. Whereas a position is a collection of tasks configured together, usually by one individual. Each position carries with it a degree of authority, accountability, and responsibility. *Authority* is the right to act or direct others. *Accountability* is the liability of task performance, and responsibility is the assignment and acceptance of a task. Organizations may be centralized or decentralized. *Centralized organizations* have board members and administrators with power and authority at the top of the organization. Decentralized organizations are just the opposite. They empower staff at all levels to make decisions and solve pressing problems. *Decentralized organizations* usually have flat structures with few hierarchical levels.

In turbulent environments, such as health care, decentralized structures are efficient and effective because they respond rapidly to environmental change. Nurse administrators must continually examine the structure and process in order to manage resources effectively and expedite the work of the organization. One method of modifying the structure is called restructuring. *Restructuring* is modifying the existing structural components of an organization; whereas *reengineering*, another method, is a renovation of the processes used to accomplish goals. Changing the structure of nursing organizations is essential to stay competitive and provide community-based care to clients through integrated health care systems. In the past, the health care service industry has not operated as a business.

Today, health care is big business and must be responsive to cost and quality issues and changing reimbursement patterns. Organizational structures provide a framework for the division of labor and the accomplishment of work. The three types of organizations are bureaucracy, matrix, and adhocracy. These organizational types can be viewed on a continuum with the classic bureaucracy on one end and the delegated organizational type adhocracy on the opposite end.

A *bureaucracy* is a tall, pyramidal, hierarchical structure where the power is centralized at the top. In a pyramidal structure, the decision makers are at the top, and the workers are at the bottom. Line positions are those that are in the chain of command and who directly contribute to the product or service of the organization. The strategic apex is another term used to denote the top decision maker positions. The operating core are the workers and the middle line managers coordinating the work. Technocrats are individuals who design, plan, change, or train people to do the work. Support staff provide services to enhance the technocrats productivity.

A *matrix structure* is used for complex work environments. It is a combination of bureaucracy and project teams. In a matrix structure, single individuals may report to two or more individuals and be evaluated by them on specific components of their work. This structure is complicated, and requires coordination and careful evaluation. The advantages include maximizing the use of specialists and interdisciplinary teamwork. Its disadvantages include the need for time-consuming activities such as monitoring and evaluating multiple project teams and individuals and for ensuring optimal productivity from groups.

Adhocracies are used when highly specialized professional groups practice together. Little supervision is needed, and individual workers are assigned to project teams to complete work.

There are five basic organizational types ranging from the most simple to the more complex. The simple structure has a wide span of control, minimal or no middle line, and no staff. The organization is typically small and new with few guidelines. A machine bureaucracy is an elaborate structure of administrative and support personnel, large units, and a pyramidal hierarchy. A professional bureaucracy has a flat structure, with few midlevel managers, but a large support staff to assist professional workers. A divisionalized form is a collection of quasi-autonomous units with a central administration. An adhocracy is a highly organic form composed of professional workers who elect to manage themselves and a flat administrative structure.

An *organizational chart* is used to graphically display the formal structure for an organization. The formal structure depicts the formal communication channels—who reports to whom and the levels of authority. The informal structure is a network within an organization that is typically oral in nature, and composed of friends and co-workers who share information. The organizational chart depicts vertical or horizontal structures. Vertical structures show how tall or centralized an organization is, and horizontal structures refer to flat or decentralized organizations.

Nursing leaders are faced with a complex, turbulent, and constantly changing health care environment to manage. They are challenged to respond to client needs and health care issues. Four major leadership initiatives to cope with health care changes are downsizing management, decentralizing support services, centralizing supply distribution, and organizing labor around technology.

Nurses who lead their organizations to success will also use new or reconfigured hospital structures. The trends noted by responsive leadership teams are flattened organizations, fluid structures, outcomes orientation, redefined staff functions with managerial accountability, reduced staff costs, subcontracting services, and refocusing on the core business. Work design, restructuring, and reengineering are all strategies to reposition a health care agency in a competitive manner. Layoffs, downsizing, and substitution of assistants for RNs are only short-term solutions for the cost concerns of managers. Nursing leaders must take a proactive stance and provide a vision for the organization, one that combines cost and quality into an efficient, effective health care system that is grounded in positive client outcomes.

LEARNING TOOLS

Group Activity: Understanding Organizational Structure

Purpose: To gain a clear understanding of the purpose and function of organizational structures.

Directions: Develop an interactive site with peers for the purpose of exchange information and ideas about organizational structure. Appoint an interactive leader who posts the discussion topic or question. Establish a timeframe—perhaps five days—where each individual contributes information and comments regarding the posted topic. Through this interactive site, valuable information and research articles about organizational structure can be shared. The interactive leader should summarize the major points in the discussion and then post the next topic for discussion.

Organizational Structure Topic Guide

1. Discuss the importance of organizational structure for work, power, and control elements.
2. Structure creates an environment in which practice takes place. Describe nursing administrators', nurse managers', and clinical nurses' roles in changing the organizational structure to improve client outcomes.
3. What type of an organizational structure works best in a turbulent, changing health care environment?
4. Describe activities nurses can use to create a positive work environment.

Group Activity: Organizational Chart Analysis

Purpose: To analyze an organizational chart in order to determine the channels of communication, staff and line positions, centralized versus decentralized structure, and a pyramidal or flat structure.

Directions: Review the organizational chart illustrated below. Either individually or in a small group, complete an organizational chart analysis by completing the study guide questions listed below.

Study Guide Questions for an Organizational Chart Analysis

1. Is this a pyramidal or flat organizational structure?
2. Are communication channels simple or complex?
3. Are there any staff positions? If so, what are they?
4. How many levels are in the hierarchy?
5. Is this a centralized or a decentralized chart?

(Once the study guide is completed, review your answers with the study guide analysis located on page 139.)

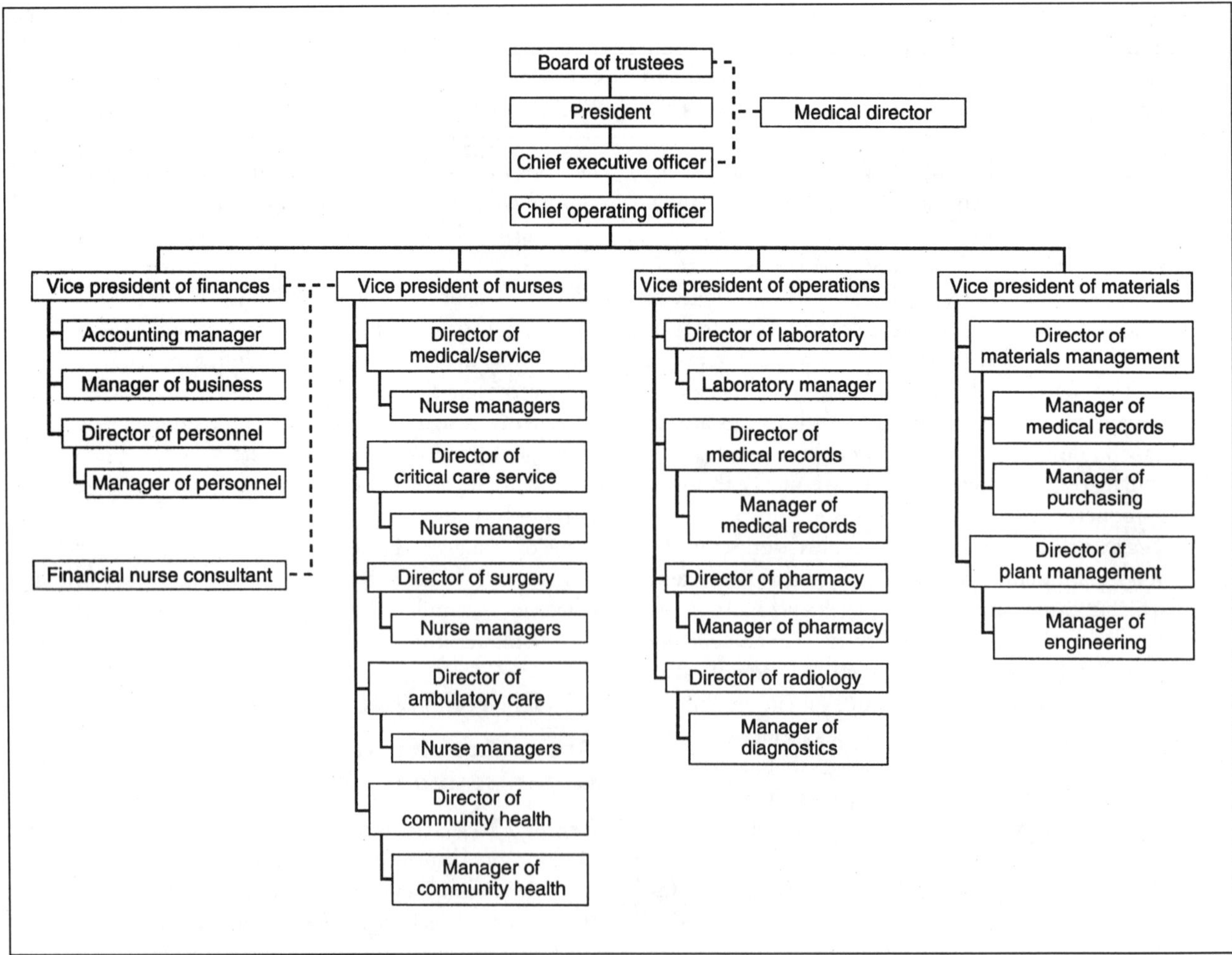

Figure 26–1. Hospital Organizational Chart

Hospital Organizational Chart Answers:

This is a pyramidal organizational structure with seven levels in the hierarchy. The communication channels are complex with a detailed reporting structure. It appears to be a very centralized organizational structure because of the multiple levels. There are two identified staff positions, the medical director and the financial nurse consultant.

CASE STUDY: ORGANIZATIONAL STRUCTURE

Jo is a nurse manager of a 45-bed surgical unit with a position control of 58 FTEs, and which currently employs 65 individuals. Christa is the nurse educator assigned to the surgical unit. Christa works with all of the surgical units since she is a clinical nurse specialist whose focus is surgical care. Jo and Christa work well as a team and they establish annual goals together and meet monthly to review progress. Jo's task is to be responsible for the fiscal and human resource management, and Christa's responsibilities include the education of new and existing employees.

Case Study Questions

1. Is Jo in a line or staff position? Is Christa in a line or staff position? What is the difference between line and staff positions?
2. For what tasks is Jo held accountable? For what tasks is Christa held accountable?
3. Who has the authority to make decisions for the surgical unit?
4. Which resources can Jo and Christa consult to determine their level of accountability?

CASE STUDY: CENTRALIZED/ DECENTRALIZED STRUCTURE

Sylvia is a vice president of a 720-bed acute care facility in New York. The hospital has been having severe financial problems because of the changes in reimbursement. Sylvia has met with the chief executive officer (CEO) and the chief financial officer (CFO) who both want immediate action to get the bottom line in the black. Since Sylvia has the largest budget with the largest number of FTEs she is asked to make all the cuts in her department. The CEO and CFO suggested layoffs, hiring assistive unlicensed personnel, and merging units to decrease the number of nurse managers in the hospital. They are not telling Sylvia what to do, however. If she can think of other cost cutting strategies, she is free to use them. (Sylvia leaves the meeting rather somber.)

Case Study Questions

1. What should Sylvia do?
2. Will the suggestions that the CEO and CFO made solve all Sylvia's problems and save money for the hospital?
3. Are the suggestions that the CEO and CFO made long-term or short-term strategies?
4. What other strategies could be employed to cut costs?

LEARNING RESOURCES

Discussion Questions

1. In turbulent environments, is a centralized or decentralized structure best for accomplishing the work of the organization? Provide a rationale for your answer.
2. What are some methods nurse administrators can use to change the structure in order to deliver high-quality care to clients?
3. Describe the five basic mechanisms that organizations use to coordinate their work.
4. What is the role of the board in an organization? How can clinical nurses impact board-level decisions?
5. What is the difference between restructuring and reengineering? Give an example of each.
6. Are there differences between the health care service industry and the private business sector?
7. What type of organizational structure would be best for a highly complex, turbulent, health care environment that employees specialists?
8. What is the difference between centralized and decentralized organizations?
9. Describe the difference between a line and a staff position. Provide an example of each.
10. When would a matrix structure for an organization be useful? What are the advantages and disadvantages of a matrix structure?

Study Questions

Matching: Write the letter of the correct response in front of each term.

_____ 1. Line position
_____ 2. Staff position
_____ 3. Authority
_____ 4. Accountability
_____ 5. Responsibility
_____ 6. Scalar process
_____ 7. Span of control
_____ 8. Reengineering
_____ 9. Centralized
_____ 10. Decentralized

A. The creation of levels of authority in a hierarchy
B. The number of workers supervised by a manager
C. A position that provides expertise and knowledge for accomplishing organizational goals
D. The right to act or direct others

_____ 11. Bureaucracy
_____ 12. Matrix
_____ 13. Adhocracy
_____ 14. Pyramidal
_____ 15. Technostructure
_____ 16. Support staff
_____ 17. Operating core
_____ 18. Horizontal structure
_____ 19. Machine bureaucracy
_____ 20. Divisionalized form

E. The liability associated with task performance
F. The allocation or acceptance of tasks
G. When the power to make decisions is concentrated at the top of an organization
H. When the power to make decisions is filtered down toward the individual worker
I. Direct line of hierarchical authority
J. Changing the operational process of an organization
K. A collection of semiautonomous units linked by a central administrative structure
L. A large administrative and support staff and a tall hierarchy
M. Few administrative layers between top administrators and workers
N. Those who perform the work of the organization by providing the service
O. Individuals who perform activities that enable individuals to do the direct work of the organization
P. Analysts who design, plan, change, or train people to do the work of the organization
Q. Tall, shaped with a wide base and narrow apex
R. A complex combination of a hierarchical structure with project teams
S. Tall, hierarchical, centralized structure
T. Flat, decentralized structure with project teams

REFERENCE

Mintzberg, H. (1983). *Structure in Fives: Designing Effective Organizations*. Englewood Cliffs, NJ: Prentice-Hall.

SUPPLEMENTAL READINGS

Fuss, M.A., Bryann, Y.E., Hitchings, K.S. & Foxet, M.A. (1998). Measuring critical care redesign: Impact on satisfaction and quality. *Nursing Administration Quarterly, 23(1)*, 1-14.

Hagenow, N.R. (1998). Management restructuring: The process of change. *Seminars for Nurse Managers, 6(2)*, 64-68.

Miller, E. (1999). Reengineering the role of a nurse manager in a patient-centered care organization. *Journal of Nursing Care Quality, 13(6)*, 47-56.

Nagelkerk, J. & Henry, B. (1993). Chain reaction. *Graduating Nurse*, 19-23.

O'Brien, B.L. (1998). St. Joseph's hospital and medical center: Nursing organizational structure. *Nursing Administration Quarterly, 22(4)*, 21-23.

ANSWERS TO TEXT STUDY QUESTIONS

Chapter 26—Organizational Structure (p. 494)

1. **What purposes for nursing does the structure of the organization serve?**

   Organizational structure serves to provide order, distinction, and a framework for goal attainment. As with other personnel, the purposes of organizational structure for nurses are to control behavioral variations among individuals, avoid chaos, direct the flow of information, determine employee positions, and provide an efficient work flow.

2. **What elements of organizational structure are found in nursing organizations?**

   The elements of organizational structure include division of labor, hierarchy of authority, rules and regulations that govern behavior, span of control, and lines of communication. All of these elements are present in nursing organizations.

3. **What elements are most important for nursing practice?**

   When identifying the elements of organizational structure that are important to nursing practice, you must consider what elements facilitate care delivery. Rules and regulations provide functional boundaries that govern behavior. The division of labor provides for delegation of responsibilities, and the lines of communication delineate line and staff reporting structures and direct the flow of information.

4. **What factors need to be assessed prior to changing the organizational culture?**

   An organizational structure is a significant element in the culture of an organization. Prior to initiating any type of change process, one must have a thorough understanding of the existing structure. It is essential to assess the complexity of the organization; the level of specialization of the workforce; the degree of centralization of services; and the formalization of policies, procedures, rules, and regulations.

5. **How do nurses foster or hinder restructuring?**

   Organizational restructuring changes roles, jobs, and positions in nursing, therefore it elicits both opposition and support. Opposition to restructuring is not surprising, especially with downsizing of the RN workforce and nursing management. Yet enhanced opportunities for nurses in a restructured health care environment include case management, care coordination across settings, advanced practice, and autonomous clinical practice.

6. **What changes are needed in nursing organizations? Why?**

   Traditionally, nursing organizations are bureaucratic. To be successful in a health care reform climate, nursing organizations must change to become more cost-effective, efficient, innovative, and flexible structures that respond quickly to a dynamic and turbulent environment. Nursing organizations must change or risk becoming bureaucratic relics.

7. **How are the structures of community agencies the same as (or different from) those of hospitals?**

   Due to their size and complexity, hospitals often have bureaucratic structures. The services provided may be diverse, with multiple divisional lines and levels of authority. A board of directors heads the structure in hospital organizations as it does in community agencies. Historically, hospitals have been designed to maintain an internal focus, whereas community agencies have been structured to have a more external focus. Community agencies that are linked to state and federal agencies are complex bureaucratic entities, while those linked with local government tend to be less complicated structures.

8. **What coordinating mechanisms are used in nursing and health care organizations?**

   Five basic mechanisms are used in nursing and health care organizations to coordinate their work: mutual adjustment, direct supervision, standardization of work processes, standardization of work outputs, and standardization of worker skills.

9. **How effective are the coordinating mechanisms used by nursing?**

   The effectiveness of coordinating mechanisms in nursing varies. The process of mutual adjustment or informal communication among peers for problem resolution has been used effectively since the inception of nursing practice. Direct supervision was effective prior to the advent of primary care nursing. However, during the decade of its popularity, delegation skills were lost and nurses are only now regaining them through education and experience. Nursing has been slow to standardize processes, outputs, and worker skills. Standardization efforts within organizations and national credentialing bodies are improving as demands for validation of competencies, cost containment, and quality increase.

10. How have authority, responsibility, and accountability been used in nursing practice? What feelings do they create?

Organizational authority is used to fulfill the responsibilities of a professional role in a specific job while professional authority is used to practice professional nursing. Each nurse who fulfills a position accepts responsibility to complete the work and maintains accountability for the quality and quantity of the assigned work. These three elements of professional practice may generate mixed feelings. Authority may produce feelings of power and esteem, whereas responsibility and accountability may generate feelings of uncertainty and fear.

11. Is power in nursing centralized or decentralized?

Decentralization of power in nursing has become more common over the years. Decentralized structures improve quality and lower costs by placing the decision-making authority closer to work processes. With increasing demands on health care entities to lower costs and improve quality, the trend to create infrastructures that decentralize the decision-making power in nursing will continue into the future.

Decentralization and Shared Governance

STUDY FOCUS

The Information Age has created new demands in response to the revolution of technology and information processing. Centers of excellence are able to respond to changes proactively in an efficient and effective manner empowering employees to make innovative decisions promptly. Decision-making authority in an organization is an essential component of job and professional autonomy. Decision-making power can be centralized, with a few administrators at the top, or decentralized, passing the power on to the individuals that the decision affects directly. Centralization and decentralization can be ranges on a continuum with centralization at one end and decentralization at the opposite extreme. Decisions can be viewed as either more or less centralized or decentralized. There is rarely a situation in which all decisions are exclusively centralized or exclusively decentralized. Vertical decentralization is the distribution of formal power down the chain of command, and horizontal decentralization is the distribution of formal power outside the chain of command where support staff participate in the decision-making process. (When an administration centralizes the structure, they are controlling decision making and holding power at the top of the organization. In contrast, an administration that decentralizes decision making empowers employees at all levels of the organization to participate.) *Governance* is the structure, process, and whole system by which a group functions and makes decisions.

During turbulent times, in complex environments, and with professional staff, decentralization is a useful tool to ensure that the organization stays flexible, innovative, and committed to solving complex, multidisciplinary problems. Participation in decision making at all levels fosters autonomy, accountability, and worker responsibility.

Communication to and from individuals is extremely important in decentralized organizations. Nurse administrators are experimenting with many different models of participatory decision making to empower nurses to provide quality care to clients. Shared governance is one professional practice framework that espouses an accountability-based governance structure. *Shared governance* is a system that fosters creativity and flexibility by empowering nurses to make autonomous clinical decisions through formal processes. The major nursing service components of shared governance include practice, quality, education, and peer governance.

Shared governance was first implemented in the late 1970s as a method to improve nurse satisfaction, improve retention, and enhance the recruitment of clinical nurses. Difficulties in establishing a shared governance environment commonly occur in a bureaucratic organization because of the complicated communication networks, rigid reporting structures, and elaborate policies and procedures that govern employee behavior. Another common problem in implementing shared governance is the difficulty of making a true change instead of a cosmetic or name change. It is much easier for an administration to use the terminology, but retain all authority and decision-making power.

The implementation of shared governance in an organization creates a constant tension between organizational and professional goals. Nurses exert their influence or control by clearly defining and articulating their scope and standards of practice, their nursing care delivery system, their knowledge specialization, their knowledge and resource development priorities, and their self- or peer evaluation.

Three major models of professional governance are the councilar model, the congressional model, and the administrative shared governance model. The *councilar model* has committees that are elected and have clearly defined authority and function. The councilar model typically has at least one committee on each of the following: practice, education, management, and quality improvement. The *congressional model* includes officers and an elected cabinet. It is modeled after the national government's structure. The *administrative shared governance model* divides administration and clinical into two separate components and identifies the authority for each. Committees and forums are held together, and decisions are made at the level where the actual work takes place. Both the administrative and council structure have decision-making power.

Changes in health care delivery require responsiveness to new client care demands on an ongoing basis. Clinical nurses are being held accountable for their actions and must take responsibility in designing and delivering care. Health care organizations will continue to change to maintain their viability and increase their market share, causing mergers, consolidations, multisite systems, and integrated health care networks.

Nursing leaders are challenged to restructure roles in order to decentralize authority to the point of service, empower clinical nurses, increase multitasking, develop work processes that support client-care delivery, and design new skill mixes. Three key criteria that administrators will be held accountable for include delivering care within financial resources, providing high-quality services, and satisfying consumer and provider service demands. A major leadership challenge will be to develop a culture of success in the organization. Governance issues will be fluid as innovations in integration within, between, and among organizations occur through partnering, strategic alliances, and vertical integrations.

LEARNING TOOLS

Group Activity: Analysis of Organizational Structure

Purpose: To analyze an organization in order to determine if it is a centralized or decentralized organization, and to determine if a shared governance framework is established.

Directions: Select a health care organization that you are familiar with and complete the Governance Study Guide.

Governance Study Guide

a. Where is the power in the organization?

____

b. How much authority does each manager have?

____

c. Who has what decision-making responsibility?

____

d. How many levels of hierarchy are there in the organization?

____

e. Do clinical nurses make autonomous clinical decisions?

____

f. Are clinical nurses elected or appointed to organizational committees?

____

g. Do clinical nurses participate in hiring, evaluating, and scheduling decisions?

____

h. How are clinical nurses' innovative ideas encouraged and received by administration?

____

i. How are assignments made on the nursing units?

____

Upon completion of the Governance Study Guide, design an organizational structure that facilitates employee participation. This exercise will help you determine the type of organizational structure that you are comfortable with and give you ideas about the type of work environment you might look for when seeking employment.

Remember that a more decentralized structure enables clinical nurses to participate at all levels of decision making. Communication is horizontal and vertical and innovations are encouraged.

CASE STUDY

Joyce has been a vice president of nursing at a 600-bed community hospital for 15 years. She has established a hierarchical nursing service and decides it is time to cut out some of the unnecessary organizational layers to contain costs. Joyce announces at the monthly management meeting in May that it is imperative that nursing management downsize. She says she will be consulting with several individuals to make the best possible and least painful choices. Joyce also announces that she has developed a shared governance model and provides a handout of the committee structure for the nursing service department. Joyce directs the managers to tell the employees that they are now working in a shared government environment and to solicit volunteers for the committees. Managers should submit volunteer names to the executive secretary. The secretary will notify the appropriate committee members when problems arise and arrange for them to meet.

Case Study Questions

1. Did Joyce implement a shared governance framework?
2. How is participation in decision making encouraged at all levels in the nursing department?
3. What benefits are there to espousing a shared governance framework?

LEARNING RESOURCES

Discussion Questions

1. Discuss the disadvantages and advantages of centralized and decentralized organizational structures.
2. How do changes in health care influence the type of governance model a hospital will choose to implement?
3. Compare and contrast the three major types of governance models.
4. What is meant by "only a cosmetic change occurred when shared governance was implemented"?
5. What is the clinical nurse's role in a shared governance model?

Study Questions

True or False: Circle the correct answer.

T F 1. The congressional model uses a council format and separates the clinical and administrative tracts.

T F 2. The administrative model elects a president and cabinet of officers who represent each nursing unit.

T F 3. The councilar model is composed of councils with elected positions.

T F 4. All clinical nurses are in favor of a shared governance system where accountability and decision making are encouraged.

T F 5. Implementation of shared governance systems is costly and requires considerable time and effort.

T F 6. Nurse leaders are challenged to design effective delivery systems in multihospital systems and integrated networks.

T F 7. Centralization is the concentration of decision-making authority at the top of the organization.

T F 8. Decentralization is dispersing decision-making authority throughout the organization.

T F 9. An organization is either centralized or decentralized.

T F 10. Savvy administrators will decentralize during crisis and centralize during stable times.

SUPPLEMENTAL READINGS

Gavin, M. Ash, D., Wakefield, S. & Wroe, C. (1999). Shared governance: Time to consider the cons as well as the pros. *Journal of Nursing Management, 7(4)*, 193-200.

Hess, R.G. (1998). Measuring nursing governance. *Nursing Research, 47(1)*, 35-42.

Johnson, K. & Schubring, L. (1999). The evolution of a hospital-based decentralized case management model. *Nursing Economics, 17(1)*, 29-35.

King, C. & Koliner, A. (1999). Understanding the impact of power in organizations. *Seminars for Nurse Managers, 7(1)*, 39-46.

Pearson, M.A. (1998). Shared governance and motivation: Planning for success. *Journal of Shared Governance, 4(2)*, 9-10.

ANSWERS TO TEXT STUDY QUESTIONS

Chapter 27—Decentralization and Shared Governance (p. 512)

1. **What is the relationship between decentralization and shared governance?**

   Decentralization occurs when the decision-making power is dispersed to many points within the organization. A shared governance model falls under the auspices of decentralization. It is one form of a professional practice model in which decision-making power is shared among staff nurses and management.

2. **How are shared governance and structure related?**

   Although shared governance may assume different forms, it is an organizational structure. It legitimizes staff nurses' influence on the administrative decision-making process.

3. **What conditions in the facility in which you are a student or employee would facilitate shared governance?**

   To identify conditions that facilitate shared governance, consider the factors that empower staff nurses to make autonomous client care decisions. Possible conditions that might be present include administrative support; interdisciplinary collaboration and team building; and educational offerings that prepare staff for authority, accountability, and resource management. A staff that is knowledgeable of the financial management processes of the organization and is encouraged to take an active role in the implementation of its strategic plan also facilitates the development of shared governance. What other conditions can you identify?

4. **Are decentralization and shared governance characteristic of current hospital nursing organizations? Current community health and long-term care organizations?**

   The last decade has seen a movement toward decentralization in hospital nursing organizations. Hospitals have been the trendsetters among health care organizations to establish more participative management structures. Many institutions have implemented models of shared governance, with varying degrees of nurse autonomy and authority over practice and processes. As integrated health care systems continue to develop, shared governance frameworks will continue to emerge in community-based environments and long-term care settings.

5. **Does changing to a shared governance model change nurses' roles? If so, how?**

   Nurses' roles in a shared governance model are expanded to accept more responsibility and accountability for decision making. Nurses will not only be expected to provide professional care, but will be instrumental in decision-making processes that affect their practice, the professional environment, and care delivery. Decisions about the acquisition and allocation of resources, educational opportunities, peer review, and quality improvement processes are examples of additional responsibilities that are a part of a shared governance model.

6. **What is the governance structure of the nursing organization with which you are the most familiar?**

   To answer this question, think about who makes the decisions in your organization. Are staff nurses involved in decisions that affect professional practice or their work environment? Is decision making mutually shared with management or is it exclusive to either management or staff? Is the scope of decision making limited to the unit or are division-level decision-making opportunities available with input to the executive decision-making body? If a shared governance model were to be identified, would it be classified as a councilar model, a congressional format, or an administrative shared governance model?

7. **What questions should be asked to determine how decentralized an organization is in reality?**

   Some questions that will assist in the determination of where the decision making power lies include: Who has the authority to make resource allocation decisions? Who makes care management decisions? To what extent do nonmanagers have power over decision-making processes? What are the lines of communication in the organization?

Models of Care Delivery

STUDY FOCUS

The assignment of nursing care personnel to clients is a basic function in a health care system. An *assignment* is the transfer of a task and the accountability for the resulting outcome (Barter & Furmidge, 1998). *Delegation* is the transfer of an assignment from a registered nurse to an assistant. The determination of the structure and method by which assignments are made are reflections of the model of care delivery. Nursing care modality or the nursing care delivery system of the organization is important in the allocation of resources and in the control of decision making about client care. The type of care modality determines, to a large extent, whether professional practice exists. Nursing care delivery systems are a mechanism to organize and deliver care to clients. The four basic elements of nursing care delivery systems that individuals consider when designing systems are clinical decision making, work allocation, communication, and management. The practice model links the mission statement, professionals, and clients in the delivery of care.

Selecting or designing a nursing care delivery system is a major task and requires a series of strategic decisions. The four strategic decisions needed include developing a philosophy of resource use, choosing a delivery system, developing practice expectations, and designing the role of the registered nurse. The six types of care modalities are functional, private duty, team, primary, case management and the current evolving care delivery types. Four of these—functional, team, primary, and case management—have been used in hospitals.

Private duty nursing, the oldest type of care modality, is a model in which the nurse cares for one client. This model is very positive for both the nurse and client and fosters a close relationship; however, it is very costly, and job security is low. Group nursing originated from private duty and was an attempt to decrease costs by grouping clients in a hospital ward. The clients then paid the nurse directly. Total client care also originated from private duty nursing. Total client care is a method of providing total care for a group of clients during one shift.

Functional nursing is the assignment of tasks to personnel prepared for that function. Examples of task assignments include medication administration, intravenous administration, baths, and vital signs. Functional nursing is efficient, but client and nurse satisfaction is low. Team nursing involves the coordination of care by a registered nurse (RN) that assigns work to RNs, LPNs and nurse's aides. The assigned team members provide the majority of care to their assigned clients. *Team nursing* is cost effective, and each member's skills are used. Modular nursing evolved from team nursing and clusters clients geographically with a group approach to care.

Primary nursing is the first professional practice model and designates 24-hour accountability for assigned clients from admission to discharge. The RN coordinates care and is accountable for the outcomes. The advantages to primary care include close client-nurse relationships and holistic care. However, the cost of care increases with the attention of a professional staff. Case management is the coordination, monitoring, and procuring of services for the multiple needs of clients. *Case management* may occur only in the hospital, based on populations, or across the health care cycle of the individual. Its advantages include cost effectiveness through a holistic approach to care. Case management in acute care settings is a system of client care delivery aimed at achieving client outcomes within effective and appropriate time frames and resources. Structured care methodologies are streamlined interdisciplinary tools to determine best practices, assist in standardization of care, assist with variance tracking, quality care and outcomes research (Cole & Houston, 1999). Critical paths are one method to manage the care and resources of clients through a written plan that identifies key activities and treatments necessary at prescribed time frames. Managed care originated from case management and is focused on specific client types and outcomes within fiscal and resource constraints.

The *current evolving types of care delivery systems* are mixed client care models. They are the second generation of professional practice models in nursing. The new evolving types tend to focus on costs, quality, and professional practice. The new type of care delivery models emphasize partnerships and interdisciplinary teams that are patient-centered. The new models are built around complex systems requiring knowledge workers to deliver high-quality integrated care. Various types of teams (cross-functional teams, self-directed work teams, multidisciplinary client care teams) are formed to complete the work required in a complex environment. Patient-centered care is the resources, patient care delivery system, and personnel organized to meet the patient's health care needs (Maehling, 1995). Key factors in the patient-centered approach are the cross-training and multiskilling of team members (Higginbotham, 1999).

Managers and clinical nurses are challenged to design client care delivery systems that are cost effective, provide quality care, and ensure client satisfaction. Important factors nurses must consider when designing care modalities are the staff, assignments, nursing and physician diagnoses, the reporting structure, decision-making autonomy, communication channels, and cost. Political, economic, and social forces are pressuring nurses to treat health care as a business with identifiable outcomes and client satisfaction. Nurses are challenged to restructure or design nursing care delivery systems to provide holistic, cost-effective client care.

LEARNING TOOLS

Group Activity: Understanding Nursing Care Delivery Systems

Purpose: To critically examine your philosophy of nursing and apply it to the design of a nursing care delivery system. This exercise entails designing a professional nursing care delivery system that you feel will provide top-quality, cost-effective care to satisfied consumers by workers who enjoy their work.

Directions: First determine the four strategic decisions about resource use, delivery systems, practice expectations, and the role of the RN. Questions that will help guide your decision making:

a. What is your philosophy of resource use? Should all clients have equal access to all types of equipment, procedures, medications, and supplies? Who should determine what is to be ordered for each unit and in what quantities? Should all nurses and unlicensed assistive personnel (UAPs) have access to all supplies and resources? How will human resources be distributed?
b. What existing nursing care delivery system will you use? Or will you design or restructure an existing care delivery system to better meet the needs of your client population and organization?
c. What are the practice expectations for each level of care provider? What are the practice expectations for the management team? Will you have working managers? How does nursing interface with other health care professionals in your organization? Will your nursing care delivery system foster collaboration and consultation in a multidisciplinary team approach?
d. What is the role of the RN? Will the RN be responsible for supervision, coordination, and provision of care? What will the roles of the other health care providers be? Who will delegate work and what process will be used?

Now examine the key components of practice when designing your nursing care delivery system:

a. Composition and skill mix of your staff—What skills are needed to accomplish client care activities? How will the staff be assigned to accomplish the work?
b. Nursing and physician diagnoses—What are the common medical and nursing diagnoses for your client population? How can the diagnostic needs of clients best be met?
c. Reporting procedures—How will reports be given from one shift to another? What type of report will be used? How will physicians be notified of client changes?
d. Communication channels—How will nurses, clients, physicians, and other health care workers communicate needs and changes in procedures? How will the manager communicate with all health care members? Will the communication network be written or verbal?
e. Cost effectiveness—How will supplies and equipment be used? What mechanisms will be in place to encourage cost-effective care? Will critical pathways be used?

After you have thought about all these questions, design a nursing care delivery system by either modifying an existing one or constructing your own. This exercise will help you determine what type of care delivery structure you prefer, give you ideas to share in your work environment, and force you to analyze the use of precious resources.

CASE STUDY

Mary Jo is the nurse manager of the respiratory unit in Middlesville, North Carolina. Middlesville hospital has been experiencing budgetary problems, and Mary Jo has been instructed to cut costs in human resources. Mary Jo designs a new care delivery system. She informs the staff the next morning that the unit will fill all of the empty positions with UAPs. She has made the assignments as follows: two RNs are assigned to pass medications and intravenous fluids, two LPNs are assigned to give baths, another LPN is assigned to do treatments, and one UAP is assigned vital signs, meal preparation, and transportation duties. Two RNs are floated to intensive care to work.

Case Study Questions

1. What type of care modality did Mary Jo design?
2. What are the advantages and disadvantages of this type of care delivery system?
3. What factors did Mary Jo need to consider?

LEARNING RESOURCES

Discussion Questions

1. What are the advantages and disadvantages of each of the six types of nursing care delivery?
2. What are the four common types of nursing care delivery systems used in hospitals?
3. What factors should nurses consider when designing or restructuring a care delivery system?
4. What social, political, and economic factors influence the delivery of client care? How?
5. What is the clinical nurse's role in designing care delivery systems?

Study Questions

Matching: Write the letter of the correct response in front of each term.

_____ 1. Nursing care modality
_____ 2. Private duty nursing
_____ 3. Team nursing
_____ 4. Primary nursing
_____ 5. Managed care
_____ 6. Case management
_____ 7. Functional nursing
_____ 8. Current evolving type
_____ 9. Total client care
_____ 10. Group nursing

A. A mixed model approach to provide care
B. Managing care to achieve specific client outcomes given fiscal and resource constraints
C. A system of health service delivery, coordination, and monitoring used to meet multiple service needs of clients
D. The assignment of clients to one nurse who has 24-hour accountability
E. Coordination of care with RN, LPN, and aide assignments by an RN to a group of clients
F. The assignment of tasks to either RNs, LPNs, or aides
G. When nurses provide care to one or more clients for one shift
H. When clients are grouped together and cared for by one nurse
I. When one nurse provides care to one client
J. A method of organizing and delivering care to clients

REFERENCES

Balik, B., & Muchliniski, E. (1998). The human side of change: Transition to teams. In J.A. Dienemann (Ed.), *Nursing Administration: Managing Patient Care* (2nd ed., pp. 163-175). Stamford, CT: Appleton & Lange.

Cole, L., & Houston, S. (1999). Structured care methodologies: Evolution and use in patient care delivery, *Outcomes Management for Nursing Practice, 3(2)*, 53-59.

Higginbotham, P. (1999). Teams: The essential work unit. In S.P. Smith & D.L. Flarey (Eds.), *Process-Centered Health Care Organizations* (pp. 113-117). Gaithersburg, MD: Aspen.

Maehling, J.A.S. (1995). Process reengineering: Strategies for analysis and redesign. In S.S. Blancett & D.L. Flarey (Eds.), *Reengineering Nursing and Health Care: The Handbook for Organizational Transformation* (pp. 61-74). Gaithersburg, MD: Aspen.

SUPPLEMENTAL READINGS

Carruth, A.K., Steele, S., Moffett, B., Rehmeyer, T., Cooper, C., & Burroughs, R. (1999). The impact of primary and modular nursing delivery systems on perceptions of caring behavior. *Oncology Nursing Forum, 26(1)*, 95-100.

Ebersole, P. (1998). Trends in care delivery models. *Geriatric Nursing: American Journal of Care for the Aging, 19(1)*, 6-7.

Glick, D.F. (1999). Advanced practice community health nursing in community nursing centers: A holistic approach to the community as client. *Holistic Nursing Practice, 13(4)*, 19-27.

Propotnik, T. (1998). The clinical resource management model. *Critical Care Nursing Clinics of North America, 10(1)*, 21-31.

Webster, J. & Cowart, P. An innovative professional nursing practice model. *Nursing Administration Quarterly, 23(3)*, 11-16.

ANSWERS TO TEXT STUDY QUESTIONS

Chapter 28—Models of Care Delivery (p. 532)

1. **Who has the authority to establish the nursing care delivery model for the institution?**

   The chief nurse executive has the authority to establish the nursing care delivery model for the institution. Nurse leaders and managers within the institution play a key role in the development and selection of the care delivery model. Organizations using a shared governance or other professional practice model include staff nurses in the development and selection process.

2. **How do nurses decide which nursing care delivery system to use?**

   Nurses involved in the selection of a nursing care delivery system use a systematic assessment process that considers client characteristics, available nursing resources, and organizational support. The selection of a nursing care delivery system requires the consideration of several issues including the role of the registered nurse, practice expectations, nursing interventions, staffing composition, accountability of nurses, decision making about care, end-of-shift reporting, physician prescribed care, communication, and cost-effectiveness. A nursing care delivery system must balance nurses' needs with those of clients, physicians, and organizations.

3. **Why are nursing care delivery systems being revised and restructured?**

   Nursing care delivery systems are being revised and restructured in an effort to provide quality client care that is cost effective. Restructuring must occur as a result of changing economical, social, technological, environmental, and political forces. Increased emphasis is being placed on cost containment, appropriate utilization of resources, professional nursing practice, multidisciplinary collaboration, access to care, institutional mergers, and service integration. New or modified care delivery systems are emerging to better fit with the changing social expectations and a dynamic health care delivery environment.

4. **What issues arise when the care delivery system is changed?**

   Changes in the care delivery system may threaten the balance between meeting client needs and those of the organization. Important issues surface related to the quality and cost of services, client and care provider satisfaction, and workforce composition. Other critical issues such as care provider role clarity; registered nurse preparation and delegation skills; a client-versus-task focused perspective; and the appropriate use of registered nurse skills, knowledge, and experience must be considered when the care delivery system is changed.

5. **What common themes emerge among the newest care delivery systems being developed? How do they compare to older models?**

   The newest care delivery systems attempt to reconfigure care provision within resource constraints, care needs, and current ideas about professional nursing practice.

   Contemporary care delivery systems emphasize outcomes management, multidisciplinary collaboration, accountability, a seamless continuum of care, new roles, alteration in skill mix, and new scheduling systems. In comparison to older models, newer ones are more complex, client-centered, and include a multidisciplinary team approach. Recent care delivery models emphasize the role of the professional nurse who is concerned with providing quality cost-effective care within the context of a larger organization.

6. **What care delivery system best fits a merger of hospital and community agencies, or are multiple care models needed?**

   It is not known which care delivery system best fits each setting in which nursing is practiced. However, concepts from case management and managed care models seek to integrate services provided between the hospital and community agencies. Efforts are underway to develop a care delivery system that will provide quality care in a cost-effective manner. The restructured system must emphasize the seamless continuum of care between multiple care providers in which services are client-focused rather than hospital or agency focused. Cooperation, commitment, and collaboration are necessary to actualize this change.

Population-based Care Management

STUDY FOCUS

The United States health care system has the world's premier acute care-based illness care system for those who can afford to pay or are insured. The health care of the general population is episodic, uncoordinated, expensive, and access to care is difficult for the uninsured. Almost 14% of the gross domestic product goes toward national health care expenditures (Health Care Financing Administration, 1999).

Healthy communities are the base of a strong, flourishing society. Two major forces in the 1990s brought about an emphasis on population-based care management. The two forces were a rise in managed care systems and a focus on community health promotion and disease prevention strategies generated by the *Healthy People 2000* initiative. *The Healthy People 2000* initiative, from the U.S. Department of Health and Human Services, is the federal government's attempt to improve health and quality of life of individuals and communities. The initiative is an important example of a community health program with a population-focused approach.

Population is defined as a group of individuals who have one or more personal or environmental characteristics in common (Williams, 1996). Members of a community who are defined in terms of a common characteristic are a population. *Target population* is the research-related term. *Population-based care management* is the integration and coordination of health services to a specified population. *Community* is an entity with a local base that is composed of a system of formal organizations or groups that are interdependent and function to meet a variety of collective needs (Schuster & Goepinger, 1996). Therefore, a community is a local entity, whereas a population is an aggregate with a common characteristic. *Disease management* is a comprehensive, integrated approach to care and reimbursement based on the disease's natural course. It is an intensive series of clinical processes and services across the health care continuum that manages an at-risk population to improve care and manage resources. *Demand management* is the use of self-care activities and decision support systems for clients to improve their health and well being while making appropriate use of the health care system (Peterson & Kane, 1997; Vickery & Lynch, 1995). *Community health* is meeting the collective needs of the group by problem identification and management within and between the community and society. *Compliance* is the degree to which a client initially assents to a treatment plan. *Adherence* is the degree to which a client continues a negotiated treatment. *Maintenance* is the degree to which a client continues positive health behaviors without supervision.

In the United States there is a move toward health care reform and reconfiguring health care. Research has demonstrated that to meet the needs of citizens, health care must move toward the development of community health management systems. The focus of health care will be on integrated systems in a team-oriented culture. Health care systems will rely heavily on information systems and flexible structures to provide access and provision of quality health care to communities. A population-based health needs assessment is the first step in addressing and designing community health care services.

Population-based program planning provides the foundation for assessment of communities; development of comprehensive program plans; identifying and mapping out resource needs; and designing an integrated, systematic evaluation plan. An integrated population-based program planning model has the four components of contextual analysis, implementation plan, budget, and evaluation plan (Hall, 1998). The six basic steps of community-focused care delivery planning include establishing the contract partnership, assessing, determining the nursing diagnosis of the problem, planning, implementing interventions, and evaluating interventions and outcomes. The five key methods of collecting data are informant interviews, participant observation, windshield surveys, secondary analysis of existing data, and surveys (Schuster & Goeppinger, 1996). The six criteria to establish community priorities include community awareness of the problem, community motivation to resolve it, the nurse's ability to influence problem solution, availability of relevant expertise, severity of consequences, and speed with which resolution can be achieved (Schuser & Goeppinger, 1996).

Often, *population-based risked identification* is used to help determine the best use of staff and clinical resources while determining the long-term health care needs of a population. The levels of risk include *primary* (prevention), *secondary* (early detection), and *tertiary* (management of an episode of care) (Burgess, 1999). As the population ages in the United States, health care costs of chronic conditions increase. With the increasing numbers of elderly there is a shift in the need for preventive care and chronic illness management (Coleman, 1999). The continuum of care is the well and worried well (self-directed care and primary care), the acutely ill (secondary and tertiary care), and the chronically ill (tertiary and long-term care) (Coleman, 1999). Case management is used for high-risk acute conditions, whereas disease management is used for chronic conditions.

The continuum of health services can be conceptualized as a linear, interactive line spanning prevention-oriented care to treatment-oriented care to long-term care. Critical elements of managed care include coordination and integration. Health care delivery emphasizes primary care and coordinated interdisciplinary comprehensive health and illness management. Managed health care services are a network of providers who deliver a package of services to a specific population for a negotiated prepayment. Nursing provides coordination of services, which requires collaboration and integration. Health care organizations need to respond to specific population-based needs to ensure their viability. Competencies of excellent nursing leadership in public health include political and business acumen, program leadership, and management capability.

LEARNING TOOLS

Case Study

Bonita is a registered nurse managing a large primary care nursing center that employs 14 family nurse practitioners, 6 medical assistants, 4 registered nurses, 4 clerical staff, and an x-ray technician. The nursing center was established in 1992 and has served the south side of the city. Bonita has been tracking the number of clients registered at the nursing center and notices that there is a definite flat line for new clients. Bonita reports this information at the staff meeting and discusses the need to conduct a population-based health needs assessment as part of their program planning. The team supports Bonita in her efforts and an in-depth community assessment is conducted.

Based upon the community needs assessment, Bonita uses criteria to establish priorities for problem resolution. Bonita determines that the four major health needs of the population that they serve are diabetic and hypertensive management, well child examinations, and women's health issues. Bonita reports her findings to the staff. During the meeting the staff divided themselves into four groups to design services, programs, and health seminars on the four topic areas. A marketing plan was developed and resources were set aside to address the issues.

Within six months, Bonita noticed an increase in new clients coming to the nursing center for services. She reported this finding to the staff, who made a commitment to involving the community in their program planning and interventions.

Case Study Questions

1. What actions did Bonita take to improve the nursing center's position in the health care market?
2. What is a population-based health needs assessment?
3. What is an integrated population-based program planning model?
4. What are criteria for determining community priorities?
5. What are the basic steps of population-based care planning?

LEARNING RESOURCES

Purpose: To review the components of a comprehensive population-based program plan for identification of needed resources, community support, and evaluation.

Population-Based Program Plan

Johanna is a registered nurse in a small rural community in central Pennsylvania. The community is very close. Major problems include a high poverty rate, teenage pregnancy, a high rate of high school dropouts, and alcoholism. She is an expert clinician and is well respected in the community. Johanna is involved in the parent teacher association for the local school, the women's guild at her church, and is active with the local library.

Johanna decides that she would like to institute a new community initiative on colon cancer awareness in the community. She has spoken to the church leaders and they have provided space for her to have a screening clinic. Johanna has met resistance from the city council for financial support for this project. The first screening clinic had a very poor turnout.

Directions: Complete the Population-based Program Planning Study Guide below. Review the scenario above and evaluate the components of the integrated population-based program planning model, the steps in establishing a community-based plan, and the criteria for determining community priorities. Describe why Johanna had a difficult time in implementing her community program. What might she have done to increase the likelihood of success for a community-based program?

Population Based Program Planning Study Guide

Components of an Integrated Population-based Program

1. The program has a clear contextual analysis.
2. The program has an implementation plan with time points.
3. The program has a budget for planning, implementation, and evaluation.
4. The program has a comprehensive systematic evaluation plan.

The completion of the components of an integrated population-based program assists the community with tackling priority community issues, having the resources to complete the project, and implementing an evaluation at the conclusion of the project.

Criteria for Determining Community Priorities

1. Is there high community awareness of the problem?
2. Is there community motivation to resolve the problem?
3. Does the nurse have the ability and expertise to influence problem resolution?
4. Is there expertise in the community to manage the problem?
5. What are the consequences of not solving the problem?
6. How quickly can the problem be resolved?

The more resources, community commitment, and expertise available, the greater the chance of success for resolving the issue. What is perceived as a priority in the community will have the greatest likelihood of success in implementation and resolution.

Developing a Community-based Plan

1. Was a community partnership established?
2. Was a comprehensive community assessment conducted?
3. Were community priority problem(s) determined?
4. Was a planning process established and was a comprehensive plan that included community involvement developed?
5. Was the plan implemented using time lines and responsibility points?
6. Was the interventions and outcomes evaluated based on the comprehensive plan?

By using a community-based plan that follows the nursing process there is greater potential for success. The community-based project is clearly identified; key individuals are included; and a plan, implementation schedule, and evaluation framework is established before implementation.

Discussion Questions

1. What is the continuum of health services?
2. What are competencies of excellent nursing leadership in public health?
3. What were the forces in the 1990s to bring an emphasis on population-based care management?
4. What are the definitions of compliance, adherence, and maintenance?
5. What are key methods of collecting data for population-based care planning?

Study Questions

Matching: Write the letter of the correct response in front of each term.

_____ 1. Population
_____ 2. Population-based care management
_____ 3. Community
_____ 4. Disease management
_____ 5. Demand management
_____ 6. Community health
_____ 7. Compliance
_____ 8. Adherence
_____ 9. Maintenance
_____ 10. Population-based risk identification

A. To help determine the best use of staff and clinical resources while determining the long-term health care needs of a population
B. A comprehensive, integrated approach to care and reimbursement based on the disease's natural course
C. A group of individuals who have one or more personal or environmental characteristics in common
D. An entity with a local base that is composed of a system of formal organizations or groups that are interdependent and function to meet a variety of collective needs
E. The degree that a client continues positive health behaviors without supervision
F. Meeting the collective needs of the group by problem identification and management within and between the community and society
G. The degree that a client continues a negotiated treatment
H. The use of self-care activities and decision support systems for clients to improve their health and well being while making appropriate use of the health care system
I. The degree that a client initially assents to a treatment plan
J. The integration and coordination of health services to a specified population

REFERENCES

Burgess, C.S. (1999). Managed care: The driving force for case management. In E.L. Cohen & V. DeBack (Eds.), *The Outcomes Mandate: Case Management in Health Care Today* (pp. 13-19). St. Louis: Mosby.

Coleman, J.R. (1999). Integrated case management: The twenty-first century challenge for HMO case managers, part I. *The Case Manager, 10(5)*, 28-34.

Health Care Financing Administration (HCFA). (1999). *National health expenditures, 1997* (HCFA Publication No. 03412). Washington, DC: U.S. Government Printing Office.

Peterson, K.W. & Kane, D.P. (1997). Beyond disease management: Population-based health management. In W.E. Todd & D. Nash (Eds.), *Disease Management: A Systems Approach to Improving Patient Outcomes* (pp. 305-342). Chicago: American Hospital Publishing.

Schuster, G.F. & Goeppinger, J. (1996). Community as client: Using the nursing process to promote health. In M. Stanhope & J. Lancaster (Eds.), *Community Health Nursing: Promoting Health of Aggregates, Families, and Individuals* (4th ed., pp. 289-314). St. Louis: Mosby.

Vickery, D. & Lynch, W. (1995). Demand management: Enabling patients to use medical care appropriately. *Journal of Occupational and Environmental Medicine, 37(5)*, 1-7.

Williams, C.A. (1996). Community-based population-focused practice: The foundation of specialization in public health nursing. In M. Stanhope & J. Lancaster (Eds.), *Community Health Nursing: Promoting Health of Aggregates, Families, and Individuals* (4th ed., pp. 21-33). St. Louis: Mosby.

SUPPLEMENTAL READINGS

Dudley, R.A., Rennie, D.J. & Luft, H.S. (1999). Population choice and variable selection in the estimation and application of risk models. *Inquiry, 36(2)*, 200-211.

Ketner, L. (1999). Managed care. Population management takes disease management to the next level. *Healthcare Financial Management, 53(8)*, 36-39.

Kraus, V.A. & Wood, J.M. (1998). Using population assessment methods to target disease management interventions in high-impact/low-prevalence diseases. *Journal of Care Management, 4(5)*, 11-12, 15-16, 31.

O'Connor, P.J. & Pronk, N.P. (1998). Integrating population health concepts, clinical guidelines, and ambulatory medical systems to improve diabetes care. *Journal of Ambulatory Care Management, 21(3)*, 67-73.

ANSWERS TO TEXT STUDY QUESTIONS

Chapter 29—Population-based Care Management (p. 546)

1. **Should all nurses be doing population-based care management?**

   Population-based care management integrates and coordinates health care services for a specific population. While the role of nurses includes integrating, coordinating, and advocating for individual clients, families, and groups, not all nurses are able to coordinate health care services that affect the health status of aggregates and communities. Population-based care management often requires advanced educational preparation to perform a population-based needs assessment; identify needed health services; and implement health planning, wellness, and prevention programs.

2. **How can nurses motivate others to facilitate coordination across organizations?**

   In order to minimize fragmentation, decrease adverse client outcomes, and reduce health care costs, nurses need to manage the continuum of care. Nurses can motivate others to facilitate coordination across organizations by emphasizing the positive impact that care management has on client outcomes and organizational viability. Through a collaborative, integrated process, clients receive comprehensive health and illness care, in a cost-effective delivery system.

3. **What is the role of informatics in population-based care management?**

   Informatics has an essential role in population-based care management. The data gathered during a community or population-based assessment can be incorporated into a composite database for analysis and interpretation. Information technology can be used to examine data such as demographic characteristics, vital statistics, disease incidence and prevalence, community resources, and health care provider characteristics. These data can be used to determine nursing diagnoses and to initiate program planning. Additionally, aggregate databases can be used for comparative studies and benchmarking across populations.

4. **Are community health and population-based care management really similar terms?**

   While community health and population-based care management are sometimes used interchangeably, they are not synonymous. The focus of community health nursing practice is the improvement of health within a community, in which the community is considered the client. In contrast, population-based care management is not necessarily limited to a given location. The population may be defined by geographic location, special interest, disease state, or some other common characteristic.

5. **Why don't all clients need case management?**

   Even though all clients need coordinated care, case management serves as an intervention that best meets the needs of targeted high-risk populations. Only 10 – 20% of the population is estimated to have the complex needs that require intensive intervention, surveillance, and follow-up using a case management model.

Case Management

STUDY FOCUS

Case management activities have the potential of saving money, improving effectiveness, and maintaining the quality of care (Cook, 1998). *Case management* is an interdisciplinary strategy that crosses settings and sites of health care. Case management is designed to coordinate care, decrease costs, and promote access to the appropriate type of needed services. In 1990, the Case Management Society of America, the organization that represents case managers, was founded. The case management role is one of the fastest growing roles in health care. Managed health care enjoyed increasing popularity with national concern over rising health care costs and expenditures, fragmentation of care, and lack of access to care. Health maintenance organizations have become the predominant form of health care coverage for businesses in the United States that employ more than 100 people (Beilman et al, 1998; Coleman, 1999; Tahan, 1998).

Managed care is the integration and coordination of financing and delivery of health care services (Grimaldi, 1996). Managed care terminology has been applied to a wide range of organizational structures, prepayment arrangements, negotiated discounts, and prior authorization agreements for services with a focus on lowering costs and maximizing the use of resources. The three most common managed care-related organizational structures are health maintenance organizations, preferred provider organizations, and privately managed indemnity health insurance plans. Today, managed care refers to reimbursement strategies of arrangements and organizations. A common form of managed care financial reimbursement is capitation. *Capitation* is a fixed dollar amount paid to provide a specific set of health care services that an insured client requires (Grimaldi, 1996). The typical arrangement for capitation is a payment to a health care provider for a per-member-per-month payment regardless of the amount of care required by the covered clients.

Case management is the use of client-focused strategies to coordinate care (Bower, 1992). A key component of case management is interdisciplinary collaboration. Case management encompasses coordination of services and sequencing of care for optimal outcomes using available resources. In acute care settings, case management is generally used for high-risk populations. A registered nurse is typically assigned the accountability for care management of clients with a specific diagnostic-related grouping over the entire hospitalization. Case management has also been employed in public health and by community nurses. Case management extends across the health care continuum. Disease management is a comprehensive, integrated approach to care and reimbursement based on a disease's natural course.

A *critical pathway* is a written plan that identifies key incidents that must occur at set times to achieve client outcomes within a predetermined time frame. There are many names associated with critical pathways, such as care steps, CareMap, critical paths, and coordinated care paths. Benchmarking and evidence-based practice are used when constructing critical pathways. *Benchmarks* are a frame of reference against which an organization can compare itself relative to others. When there are differences between what is expected and what actually occurs on the critical pathway, a variation results. A *variation* is a deviation from what is expected. A variation may be positive or negative.

Managed care is a broad term and can be viewed as a system that provides structure and focus for managing the use, cost, quality, and effectiveness of health services. Many disciplines lay claim to case management. The historical perspective of case management tends to be discipline-specific. Social work reports that case management began with Mary Richmond and the early settlement houses. The insurance companies' perspective is that case management began with the management of catastrophic and high-cost insurance cases. In nursing, case management began with private duty nursing. With the rise of the early settlement houses and large numbers of immigrants and poor, there was a need for coordination of health care services. Public and human services in the United States were initiated in this era. Lillian Wald and Mary Brewster, nurses who were identified as social workers, founded the Henry Street Settlement in 1895. Community service coordination was a forerunner to case management and began at the turn of the century in public health programs. The term *case management* occurred in the literature in the 1970s in social welfare literature, followed by the nursing literature.

There are many case management models in the literature. Case management exists in many contexts across many settings. Case management can be described as a system, role, technology, process, and service (Bower, 1992). There are two major nursing models identified in the literature: the New England Model of acute care nursing case management and the community-based model of Carondelet St. Mary's. There are four models in social work: broker, primary therapist, interdisciplinary team, and comprehensive.

There are four basic principles that guide nursing case management, including coordination and integration of holistic care, promotion and preservation of health, conservation and allocation of resources, and provision of follow-up care. Case management programs are based on roles and functions of case managers. Priorities for case management include a high rate of recidivism, unpredictable care needs, significant complications, comorbidities or variances in care outcomes, high-risk profiles or high-cost cases. The general process for developing a case management program includes assessment, identify high-volume or high-risk cases, determine problems with high-volume or high-risk cases and set goals, form an interdisciplinary team, design a critical pathway, develop a pilot program, and evaluate the pilot. The ten-step process for developing a case management plan includes designing the format, selecting the target population, organizing the interdisciplinary team, educating the team, examining the current process, reviewing the literature, establishing the length of the plan, developing the content, conducting a pilot study, and standardizing the plan.

Nurses have two roles: that of caregiver and care coordinator (McClure, 1991). The emphasis on managed care in integrated health systems requires a new type of clinical nursing practice system. Case management is one approach to redesigning care delivery systems. Case management is a growing trend with increasing opportunities for nurses. As shifts occur in nursing care delivery systems to case management, nurses' job responsibilities and roles will shift. A trend in case management is the push for accountability and accreditation.

LEARNING TOOLS

Case Study

Dale is a nurse manager on a 52-bed neurological unit in a large community hospital. The administration has just informed Dale that he needs to cut 15% from his budget for the upcoming year. He recently attended a case management conference that had a breakout session on critical pathways. At the conference they discussed several strategies to conserve scarce resources. Dale learned the general process for developing a case management program and has instituted these steps in order to effect change on his unit. Dale decided to form an interdisciplinary team to design a critical pathway for the highest-volume DRG clients for whom his staff provides services.

Case Study Questions

1. What is the general process for developing a case management program that Dale will use?
2. Will development of a critical pathway save resources on Dale's unit?
3. What are the steps for developing a critical pathway?
4. What criteria should Dale use for determining which critical pathway to develop?
5. Who should be involved in designing the critical pathway?

Case Study

Bob is a family nurse practitioner who works for a health maintenance organization (HMO) in Orlando, Florida. Bob is responsible for coordinating the care for a caseload of clients who enroll in the HMO. Bob's boss has told him that the objectives of his care coordination and delivery should focus on lowering costs with maximum value and quality outcomes. Bob is careful to refer clients to only those specialists listed on the preferred provider list since he knows that they have agreed to a discounted payment arrangement. Bob also provides holistic care with an emphasis on health promotion and wellness.

Case Study Questions

1. What type of care modality is Bob using at the HMO? Is it case management versus managed care?
2. What are the characteristics of case management versus managed care?
3. Can Bob refer outside of the preferred provider specialist list that the HMO provides for him?

LEARNING RESOURCES

Group Activity: Understanding Critical Pathways

Purpose: To explore the role and design of critical pathways in the delivery of health care to clients.

Directions: Divide yourselves into small groups of four. Each small group should discuss the role of critical pathways in health care delivery, determining what types of client problems/diagnoses lend themselves to critical pathway development. Select one client problem/diagnosis and sketch out a critical pathway. (Each small group should bring a critical pathway from where they work [clinic, hospital] and share it with everyone during the study session).

When each small group shares its critical pathway, compare your critical pathway with those that the hospitals or clinics where you practice use. Notice the critical steps or client points at which treatment, medical, nursing, or other health care worker intervention is required. Also note the length of time for each and the desired client outcomes. Finally, note the similarities and differences in the structure of the critical pathways among the various groups, hospitals, and clinics. Discuss and summarize these key points.

Discussion Questions

1. What was the impetus for the development of case management?
2. Compare and contrast case management and managed care.
3. What types of case management models are there in the literature?
4. What are the four basic principles that guide nursing case management and what is the general process for developing a case management program?
5. How can critical pathways be used in organizations to improve quality and decrease costs of care?
6. What are the leadership and management challenges for nurses for designing care delivery systems in the future?
7. What is the clinical nurse's role in the provision of care, coordination of care, and the design of new care delivery systems?

Study Questions

Matching: Write the letter of the correct response in front of each term.

_____ 1. Capitation
_____ 2. Critical pathways
_____ 3. Benchmark
_____ 4. Variation
_____ 5. Disease management

A. A comprehensive, integrated approach to care and reimbursement that is based on a disease's natural course
B. A frame of reference against which an organization can compare itself relative to others
C. A deviation from what is expected that may be positive or negative
D. A fixed dollar amount that is paid to provide a specific set of health care services than an insured client requires
E. A written plan that identifies key incidents that must occur at set times to achieve client outcomes within a predetermined time frame

True or False: Circle the correct answer.

T F 1. Case management is an interdisciplinary strategy that crosses settings and sites of care.

T F 2. The case manager role has been one of the slowest growing roles in health care in the last ten years.

T F 3. The process of developing and using critical paths encourages both critical thinking and accountability.

T F 4. Critical pathways can and should be individualized to clients.

T F 5. Managed care is a broader term than case management.

T F 6. Nurses must document their effects on client outcomes to demonstrate that they can provide cost-effective services.

T F 7. Case management is frequently associated with health maintenance organizations and preferred provider organizations.

T F 8. Managed care is care coordination and delivery at the provider-client level.

T F 9. Managed care typically is used for only high-priority clients.

T F 10. Critical pathways are used only with case management.

T F 11. Multidisciplinary teams are essential in a complex health care environment.

T F 12. Case management entails providing holistic care, the conservation of resources, and care across episodes and settings.

T F 13. Case management focuses on continuity of the plan.

T F 14. Registered nurses are moving from a care providing role to a care coordinating role.

REFERENCES

Beilman, J.P., Sowell, R.L., Knox, M. & Phillips, K.D. (1998). Case management at what expense? A case study of the emotional costs of case management. *Nursing Case Management, 3(2)*, 89-95.

Bower, K.A. (1992). *Case management by nurses*. Kansas City, MO: American Nurses Publishing.

Coleman, J.R. (1999). Integrated case management: The 21st century challenge for HMO case managers, part 1. *The Case Manager, 10(5)*, 28-34.

Cook, T.H. (1998). The effectiveness of inpatient case management: Fact or fiction? *Journal of Nursing Administration, 28(4)*, 36-46.

Grimaldi, P.L. (1996). A glossary of managed care terms. *Nursing Management*, Special Supplement (October), 27(10), 5-7.

McClure, M. (1991). Introduction. In I.E. Goertzen (Ed.), *Differentiating Nursing Practice: Into the Twenty-First Century* (pp. 1-11). Kansas City, MO: American Academy of Nursing.

Tahan, H.A. (1996). A ten-step process to develop case management plans. *Nursing Case Management, 1(3)*, 112-121.

SUPPLEMENTAL READINGS

Allen, N.E. & Meduna, E. (1999). Interdisciplinary care. Development and implementation of a case management model for long term care. *Journal of Gerontological Nursing, 25(8)*, 42-49.

Anderson, M.A. & Tredway, C.A. (1999). Communication: An outcome of case management. *Nursing Case Management. 4(3)*, 104-111.

Cesta, T.G. & Falter, E.J. (1999). Case management: Its value for staff nurses. *American Journal of Nursing, 99(5)*, 48-51.

Forbes, M.A. (1999). The practice of professional nurse case management. *Nursing Case Management, 4(1)*, 28-33.

Johnson, C. & Birmingham, J. (1999). How to use research information to improve case management practice. *Journal of Care Management, 5(3)*, 41-42, 44, 46.

Mathews, P. (1999). Case management information systems: How to put the pieces together now and beyond year 2000. *Nursing Case Management, 4(2)*, 80-84.

Taylor, P. (1999). Comprehensive nursing case management: An advanced practice model. *Nursing Case Management, 4(1)*, 2-13.

Tonges, M.C. (1998). Job design for nurse case managers: Intended and unintended effects on satisfaction and well-being. *Nursing Case Management, 3(1)*, 11-25.

ANSWERS TO TEXT STUDY QUESTIONS

Chapter 30—Case Management (p. 567)

1. **What are the goals of case management?**

   Case management strives to link, manage, or organize services to meet client needs in the most cost-effective manner. Essential goals of case management include coordinating client-focused care, promoting access to appropriate and needed services, and conserving and allocating scarce resources. Another important goal of case management is the provision of follow-up care that tracks and guides service delivery across time and settings.

2. **What are the goals of managed care? How do they compare to those of case management?**

   Managed care strives to lower costs and maximize the value of services and resources. Managed care goals are similar to those of case management in that both seek to reduce costs and conserve resources. Managed care differs from case management in that managed care goals are broader and provide the structure and focus for managing the use, cost, and effectiveness of health services for all clients. In contrast, case management goals focus on delivery of care for clients with highly complex or long-term health care needs.

3. **What are the outcomes anticipated by case management? By managed care?**

   Anticipated outcomes for case management are the achievement of client outcomes within effective and appropriate time frames and resources. Nurse case managers coordinate and integrate the seamless continuum of care to reduce fragmentation and redundancy. Managed care outcomes focus on cost control and resource conservation by monitoring client-care decisions and resource allocation.

4. **How is case management affecting the role of the nurse?**

   Case management is expanding the role of the nurse. Nurse case managers are responsible for the coordination and integration of multidisciplinary services across the continuum of care. Effective case management requires specialized knowledge and expertise, as well as advanced education to address the complex and diverse needs of clients.

5. **Who should be the case manager?**

   Advanced practice nurses are skilled in the coordination of client care, possessing expert knowledge, experience, and education. As such, they are imminently qualified to be case managers. Given the interdisciplinary nature of case management, the advanced practice nurse is able to draw on a wealth of knowledge to coordinate efforts of the health care team to achieve desired client outcomes.

6. **Does the public health model apply to hospital settings? Why or why not?**

   The focus of traditional public health models has been the coordination of client-centered care within the community setting. In contrast, the focus of tertiary care models has been on the treatment of acute, episodic health care conditions. As societal and economic pressures have demanded that health care organizations implement cost-effective, quality care, the hospital setting has patterned the care delivery system after the public health model.

   The perspective of the public health model guides the health care organization to coordinate and integrate services across the continuum from hospital to community, thereby reducing costs and eliminating redundancy of services.

7. **Do all clients need case management?**

   While all clients need coordinated care, case management best serves the needs of targeted, high-risk populations. All clients do not need the close monitoring that case management provides, especially in an environment where case managers are a limited resource. A recent alternative to managing the use, cost, quality, and effectiveness of health care services has been the implementation of managed care systems.

Staffing and Scheduling

STUDY FOCUS

Staffing and scheduling are key nursing leadership and management functions. These activities are complex and require considerable time. Staffing and scheduling are important components in the effective provision of cost-effective, client-centered care and in the satisfaction, retention, and recruitment of nurses. The major goal of staffing and scheduling systems is to identify the need and determine the proper type of personnel required to provide patient services (Smith, 1994). *Staffing* is the development of a plan to hire qualified workers to fill designated positions in an organization. *Scheduling* is implementing the staffing pattern to assign workers to cover specific shifts and days on specific units. *Staff mix* is the skill level of workers required to provide care. *Nursing resources* include the number and types of workers designated to provide nursing services. The *nursing workload* is a compilation of nursing care needs of clients. *Acuity* is the intensity or severity of client illness. *Nursing intensity* is the amount and complexity of care required by clients. A *nurse extender* is a worker who completes designated tasks in order to assist the nurses to care for a larger number of clients or to offer clients a broader selection of services.

Staffing decisions are complex and require planning and careful consideration for maximum effectiveness. Staffing and scheduling activities are unique to each care delivery setting. There are similarities in scheduling such as ensuring safe, cost-effective care; maximizing resources; managing workload variation; and using a variety of providers (Barratt & Schultz, 1997). Four essential elements of staffing decisions include a statement of philosophy, general objectives for the department and specific objectives for the unit, job descriptions for all skill levels, and a statement of the frequency of nursing care along with a designation of who will provide the services. Typically, staffing decisions are based on a measure of volume and/or time. Volume measures include census, visits, births, operations, and client contacts. One method of volume calculation is hours per patient day (HPPD). *HPPD* is a calculation of nursing hours needed per unit of service.

Two methods used to guide nurse staffing are fixed and variable staffing. *Fixed staffing* is a fixed maximum workload requirement. This type of staffing method is based on the assumption that one will have maximum workload conditions. *Variable staffing* is based on a supplementary approach and involves staffing below maximum workload conditions. A proposed third type of staffing method is a semiflexible system whereby 15% of the staff is fixed. In semiflexible staffing, the fixed staff are supplemented based on volume and acuity.

There are eleven steps in designing a staffing pattern. First, select criteria to determine the intensity levels of clients or units of service. Second, determine the time required to complete the work. The third step is to collect data to determine the validity of a set classification system. Fourth, collect sufficient data (type and quantity) to evaluate your proposed staffing method. Fifth, determine the average number of minutes per activity or task. The sixth step is to establish a performance time for new functions. Seventh, decide on the staff mix necessary to complete the work. Eighth, determine the amount of time per client type necessary (severity of illness) for each skill level. Ninth, establish a projected unit of service projection for the year. The tenth step is to calculate the total number of nursing hours and the number of individuals by skill mix that will be needed per year. Finally, designate the number of individuals per shift each day and their skill mix. Include a calculation for time off and administrative activities.

Many types of client classification systems are in use today. The three broad types of client classification systems include prototype, factor, and computerized real-time factor. A prototype client classification system is designed to categorize clients by broad categories and characteristics. The factor client classification system uses critical indicators to determine individual care needs. In the factor systems, allowances are made for the indirect care activities required. The computerized real-time factor systems are based on actual care requirements for individual clients.

Differentiated nursing practice is a philosophy of nursing roles, functions, and work based on education, experience, and competence. Four tiers of differentiated practice are general health care aides, nurse professionals who handle emerging patterns, nurse professionals who handle complex changes, and nurse professionals who develop a knowledge base. The educational preparation of nurses is diverse ranging from a diploma to a baccalaureate degree. The use of nurse extenders (NEs) has created much controversy in the nursing profession. As hospitals redesign and restructure client-centered delivery care systems, the number and role of nurse extenders has expanded. There are concerns that nurse extenders are not adequately trained to perform multiple tasks and therefore compromise quality care.

Managing human resources is an important leadership and management function as personnel costs are the single largest health care expense item in an organization's operating budget. During the mid 1980s, DRGs and prospective reimbursement were introduced, and during the mid 1990s, health care reform and restructuring occurred in the midst of economic pressures. Layoffs, downsizing, and restructuring created short-term economic gains. Staffing experimentation and redesign were introduced to reduce health care costs. Job uncertainty, low morale, mandatory overtime, and increased workload requirements triggered unionization efforts and concern regarding client safety.

LEARNING TOOLS

Activity: Staffing and Scheduling

Purpose: To become familiar with the staffing and scheduling process.

Introduction: Staffing a unit in a hospital or ambulatory care clinic is a challenging process. A manager must assess employees' requests for time off which include vacation, scheduled days off, and personal time. They must also handle the call-ins for sick time. To effectively staff a unit, the manager must establish a skill-mix level and project a unit service figure. The activity below provides you an opportunity to staff a unit and see the complexities of scheduling and staffing.

Staffing and Scheduling Scenario:

B6-Oncology unit (25 beds)
Average daily census: 17
Skill mix: 75% RNs
25% NEs

The nurse manager has determined that 10 staff are required for a 24-hour period. The nurse manager must cover 24 hours per week for 7 days a week. The breakdown for % of nurses needed is: days–45%, evening–36%, and nights–19%.

Employees: RNs: Susie is full-time (7-3); Jen is full-time (7-3); Jon is full-time (7-3); Sylvia is full-time (7-3); Ben is full-time (7-3 and 3-11); Jake is full-time (3-11); Kim is full-time (3-11); Cindy is 24 hours per week (3-11); Jack works on an as-needed (prn) basis (3-11 and 11-7); Tom is full-time (11-7); and Jan is full-time (11-7).

NEs: Jill is full-time (7-3); Joan is 24 hours per week (7-3); Jeremy is prn (3-11); Jerry is part-time 24 hours per week (3-11); Janet is prn (3-11); and Jessie is 32 hours per week (11-7). It is important to hire some prn or pool nurses who are flexible to assist in meeting vacation coverage.

RN requests: Susie cannot work Mondays because of school. Jen is getting married and needs September 1-17 off for her honeymoon. Jon is going away for a fishing trip and needs the first weekend of September off. Jack does not want to work Tuesdays and Thursdays because of babysitting difficulties and does not want every weekend.

NE requests: Jessie will be on vacation September 1-10. Janet will not be able to work Fridays because of a continuing education course.

Directions: Create a schedule with the following requests using the census of 17, and calculate the number of staff needed per shift. First determine how many employees are on each shift—day, evening, and night shifts. Then calculate the number of RNs and NEs needed per day, evening, and night shifts. Next, put all the requests on your calendar. Finally, create a schedule, using the empty schedule grid on the following page (remember, employees do not like working every weekend).

Questions to Consider

1. How many employees will be scheduled for each shift?
2. What type of employees will be scheduled for each shift? How many of each skill level?
3. Are there any vacation or personal requests?
4. Who works full time and who works part time? What are the part-time employees' hours?

SCHEDULE FOR SEPTEMBER 2000

September 7–3 Shift

	F	S	S	M	T	W	TH	F	S	S	M	T	W	TH	F	S	S	M	T	W	TH	F	S	S	M	T	W	TH	F	S
	1	2	3	4	5	6	7	8	9	10	11	12	13	14	15	16	17	18	19	20	21	22	23	24	25	26	27	28	29	30
RNs Susie (FT)																														
Jen (FT)																														
Jon (FT)																														
Sylvia (FT)																														
Ben (FT)																														
NEs Jill (FT)																														
Joan (PT)																														
Jeremy (PRN)																														

September 3–11 Shift

RNs Jake (FT)																														
Kim (FT)																														
Cindy (FT)																														
NEs Jerry (PT)																														
Janet (PRN)																														

September 11–7 Shift

RNs Tom (FT)																														
Jan (FT)																														
Jack (PRN)																														
NEs Jessie (PT)																														

Summary: Working with staffing and scheduling is complex. When people call in due to illness or personal crisis, finding an individual to fill the opening may be harrowing. Meeting individual requests in a tight schedule can be problematic. Many units have resorted to self-scheduling to give staff more flexibility to plan their work and personal lives and to encourage them to cover each other's shifts.

One Possible Solution: There should be 5 staff on 7-3, 3 on 3-11, and 2 on 11-7. Next, calculate how many RNs and NEs should be scheduled per shift. On 7-3, there should be 4 RNs/1 NE; on 3-11 there should be 2 RNs/1 NE; and on 11-7 there should be 1 RN/1 NE. Nurse managers have the flexibility to shift the total number of RNs and NEs within the 24-hours shift, and at times, they may alter the skill mix throughout the year to cover vacations and requests. The key is to keep salaries averaging out over the year (remember, a nurse manager budgets salaries based on the number of RNs and NEs working per shift). Many times, weekends are typically staffed with fewer nurses in order to allow staff members every other weekend off. Following is a sample of a completed schedule based on the situation described.

SCHEDULE FOR SEPTEMBER 2000

September 7–3 Shift

	F	S	S	M	T	W	TH	F	S	S	M	T	W	TH	F	S	S	M	T	W	TH	F	S	S	M	T	W	TH	F	S
	1	2	3	4	5	6	7	8	9	10	11	12	13	14	15	16	17	18	19	20	21	22	23	24	25	26	27	28	29	30
RNs																														
Susie (FT)	7-3	7-3	7-3	X	X	7-3	7-3	X	7-3	7-3	X	7-3	7-3	7-3	7-3	X	X	X	7-3	7-3	7-3	X	7-3	7-3	X	7-3	7-3	7-3	7-3	X
Jen (FT)	VAC	X	X	VAC	VAC	VAC	VAC	VAC	X	X	VAC	VAC	VAC	VAC	VAC	X	X	7-3	7-3	7-3	X	7-3	7-3	7-3	7-3	X	X	7-3	7-3	7-3
Jon (FT)	7-3	X	X	7-3	7-3	7-3	X	7-3	7-3	7-3	7-3	X	7-3	7-3	7-3	X	X	7-3	7-3	7-3	X	7-3	7-3	7-3	X	7-3	7-3	7-3	7-3	X
Sylvia (FT)	7-3	7-3	7-3	X	7-3	7-3	7-3	7-3	X	X	7-3	7-3	7-3	X	7-3	7-3	7-3	7-3	7-3	X	7-3	7-3	X	X	7-3	7-3	7-3	X	7-3	7-3
Ben (FT)	X	3-11	3-11	7-3	7-3	X	7-3	X	7-3	7-3	3-11	X	7-3	7-3	7-3	7-3	7-3	X	X	7-3	7-3	X	7-3	7-3	7-3	7-3	X	7-3	7-3	3-11
NEs																														
Jill (FT)	7-3	7-3	7-3	7-3	X	X	7-3	7-3	7-3	X	7-3	7-3	X	7-3	7-3	7-3	7-3	X	7-3	7-3	7-3	7-3	X	X	7-3	7-3	7-3	7-3	X	7-3
Joan (PT)	7-3	7-3	7-3	7-3	X	X	7-3	7-3	X	7-3	7-3	7-3	7-3	X	X	7-3	7-3	7-3	X	X	7-3	X	X	X	7-3	X	X	X	X	7-3
Jeremy (PRN)	X	X	X	7-3	7-3	7-3	X	7-3	7-3	7-3	7-3	X	X	7-3	X	X	X	7-3	X	X	X	7-3	X	X	X	X	7-3	X	X	X

September 3–11 Shift

RNs																														
Jake (FT)	3-11	X	X	3-11	3-11	3-11	X	3-11	3-11	3-11	X	3-11	3-11	3-11	3-11	X	X	3-11	3-11	3-11	X	3-11	3-11	3-11	X	3-11	3-11	3-11	3-11	X
Kim (FT)	3-11	3-11	3-11	X	3-11	3-11	3-11	3-11	X	X	3-11	3-11	X	3-11	3-11	3-11	3-11	X	3-11	3-11	3-11	3-11	X	X	3-11	3-11	X	3-11	3-11	3-11
Cindy (FT)	X	X	X	3-11	3-11	X	3-11	3-11	3-11	3-11	X	3-11	3-11	3-11	3-11	X	X	3-11	3-11	3-11	3-11	X	3-11	3-11	3-11	X	3-11	3-11	3-11	X
NEs																														
Jerry (PT)	3-11	X	X	3-11	X	3-11	X	X	3-11	3-11	X	X	3-11	X	X	X	X	3-11	X	X	3-11	X	3-11	3-11	X	3-11	3-11	X	X	X
Janet (PRN)	X	3-11	3-11	X	7-3	7-3	3-11	X	X	X	3-11	X	X	X	X	3-11	3-11	X	X	X	X	X	X	X	3-11	X	X	X	X	3-11

September 11–7 Shift

RNs																														
Tom (FT)	11-7	X	X	11-7	11-7	11-7	11-7	X	11-7	11-7	11-7	X	11-7	11-7	11-7	X	X	11-7	11-7	11-7	11-7	X	11-7	11-7	11-7	X	11-7	11-7	11-7	X
Jan (FT)	11-7	11-7	11-7	X	11-7	11-7	11-7	11-7	X	X	11-7	11-7	X	11-7	11-7	11-7	11-7	X	11-7	11-7	11-7	11-7	X	X	11-7	11-7	X	11-7	11-7	11-7
Jack (PRN)	X	11-7	11-7	11-7	X	X	X	11-7	11-7	11-7	X	X	X	X	X	X	X	X	X	X	X	3-11	X	X	X	X	X	X	X	11-7
NEs																														
Jessie (PT)	VAC	X	X	VAC	VAC	VAC	VAC	VAC	X	X	X	11-7	11-7	X	X	11-7	11-7	11-7	X	X	X	11-7	11-7	11-7	X	11-7	11-7	X	X	X

CASE STUDY

Dorothy, a graduate-prepared nurse manager of a 79-bed medical unit, decides to operationalize differentiated nursing practice in order to maximize the use of each nurse's skills and knowledge base. The medical unit is staffed by nurse's aides; licensed practical nurses; and diploma-, associate degree-, baccalaureate-, and graduate-prepared nurses. Dorothy conducts a literature review to obtain pertinent information and to review successful models of differentiated nursing practice. Then Dorothy seeks volunteers to form a task force to modify job descriptions and examine compensation levels for differentiated practice.

Case Study Questions

1. Is it possible to establish a staffing plan based on a differentiated practice model?
2. What might be the basis for differentiating practice?
3. Is it appropriate to compensate nurses based on differentiated practice? If so, why? If not, why not?

LEARNING RESOURCES

Discussion Questions

1. What factors make staffing and scheduling complex?
2. Should clinical nurses be given the opportunity to assist in scheduling? If so, why? If not, why not? Should there be scheduling parameters established by the administration? Or should clinical nurses establish their own scheduling guidelines?
3. How do you calculate HPPD? Is this a useful calculation?
4. What must be considered when developing a patient classification system?
5. What are the three broad types of patient classification and what are the differences and similarities among them?

Study Questions

True or False: Circle the correct answer.

T F 1. Staffing is the implementation of a staffing pattern indicating the number and type of workers to be scheduled per shift.

T F 2. Variable staffing is based upon a set maximum workload requirement.

T F 3. Client classification is the grouping of clients according to nursing care requirements.

T F 4. Differentiated nursing practice uses criteria such as education, experience, and competence.

T F 5. Restructuring has enhanced nursing practice and increased the need for RNs in hospitals.

T F 6. Nurse extenders assist nurses to perform client care tasks including vital signs and assessments.

T F 7. Acuity is the severity of a client illness.

T F 8. Components in determining the severity of illness include client dependency, complexity, the time to complete tasks, and the skill level of the worker needed.

T F 9. Staffing decisions are based solely on an individual's philosophy.

T F 10. Nursing workload is the number of client days and the hours of nursing care required per client day.

SUPPLEMENTAL READINGS

Blegen, M.A., Goode, C.J., & Reed, L. (1998). Nurse staffing and patient outcomes. *Nursing Research, 47(1)*, 43-50.

Hollabaugh, S. & Kendrick, S. (1998). Staffing: The five-level pyramid. *Nursing Management, 29(2)*, 34-36.

Kirby, M.P., Dkost, P., Holdwick, C.C., Poskie, M., Glaser, D. & Sage, M. (1998). Improving staffing with a resource management plan. *Journal of Nursing Administration, 28(11)*, 25-29.

Ferriell, K.M., Sutton, K., Fisher, A., Rosen, J., Allen, B., Geist, M., Hewlett, K.C., Mangrum, D., Vondette, J., Jones, C., & Reese, S.M. (1999). Managers forum. Staffing standards...I know that no national standard exists for staffing an emergency department because so many different factors must be considered. How are other departments justifying staffing needs? *Journal of Emergency Nursing, 25(3)*, 216-227.

Waters, A. (1999). New rostering system will calculate safe staffing levels. *Nursing Standards, 13(46)*, 7.

ANSWERS TO TEXT STUDY QUESTIONS

Chapter 31—Staffing and Scheduling (p. 588)

1. **Should nursing services be staffed to the minimum, maximum, or mean? Why?**

   Staffing and scheduling decisions are a challenging yet critical component of the nurse management role. Two general frameworks used to determine staffing include traditional fixed staffing and controlled variable staffing. The traditional fixed staffing model is based on fixed projected maximum workload requirements and workload conditions, using historical census trend data and projections. The controlled variable staffing method is built below maximum workload conditions, with staffing supplementation as needed. While unique factors may influence staffing and scheduling decisions based on the care delivery context, there are similar factors considered across settings: ensuring safe, cost-effective care; dealing with workload fluctuations; using a variety of caregivers; and implementing effective, responsible resource management.

2. **What is the influence of the budget on staffing and scheduling?**

   The budget is a major influential factor in the development of staffing and scheduling plans. Current economic constraints and limited financial resources have resulted in intense scrutiny of personnel costs and use. The nursing personnel salaries account for a significant proportion of a health care organization's operating budget. In response to current economic pressures, cost reduction strategies include strict staffing plans, nursing personnel layoffs, and the introduction of unlicensed assistive personnel.

3. **To what extent should staff preferences determine staffing and scheduling?**

   Staffing and scheduling is a critical core function for nurse managers that require a balance between competing interests and needs. Predetermined standards, budget constraints, personal preferences, and legal aspects must all be taken into consideration. Staff satisfaction with scheduling is important, especially with varied shift lengths and unorthodox work hours as nurses attempt to meet the demands of their personal lives. A negotiation process may occur to ensure that both organizational and personal needs are met.

4. **What is the role of the patient classification system for staffing and scheduling?**

   The patient classification system provides a quantified measure of nursing time and effort required to care for clients. It attempts to identify patient acuity to use as a proxy for workload, which becomes the basis for staffing and scheduling decisions. There are three broad types of patient classification systems: prototype, factor, and computerized real-time factor systems, all of which have been criticized concerning their reliability, validity, and comparability across settings. Other issues with patient classification systems are related to impracticality of some systems, the time involvement necessary for development and maintenance, and the inability to evaluate generated data for usefulness to nursing and the organization.

5. **Should a manager do the schedule or should staff schedule themselves?**

   Scheduling methods vary and are setting-specific. Scheduling decisions may be limited to nursing personnel and staff, as well as managers and unit secretaries. Scheduling methods may involve computerized scheduling, managerial scheduling, self-scheduling, or a combination of some or all methods. No matter what scheduling method is selected, use of a consensus building process will facilitate meeting hours of care delivery and organizational financial goals. In a shared governance environment, a self-scheduling method may reflect autonomous practice, participation in decision making, and administrative support.

6. **What is the "right" mix of RNs and assistive personnel?**

   It is not clear what the effective and efficient mix of RNs and unlicensed assistive personnel is or should be. Experimentation is occurring with reconfigurations of personnel, differentiated practice, and the introduction of assistive personnel. Empirical and evaluative efforts have been minimal and without sufficient rigor to document the effect of nurse extenders in health care. It is important that nurses examine the use of nurse extenders and their impact using cost, satisfaction, and quality indicators.

Data Management and Informatics

STUDY FOCUS

Accurate and timely data are essential to make decisions about client care and organizational management (Newbold, 1998). Computer applications in nursing administration are tools to make effective decisions to enhance quality client care. Nursing must develop or use existing standardized nursing databases to make meaningful comparisons across clinical sites. Computer applications have provided an efficient and effective method of acquiring financial data to evaluate outcomes of care.

Computers are the tools for managing data. *Informatics* is a combination of computer and information science. *Nursing informatics* is the management of nursing data, information, and knowledge as it is applied to nursing care delivery. *Effectiveness research* is the use of large data sets applying epidemiological methods to evaluate relationships. *Management information systems* (MIS) are integrated to collect, store, retrieve, and process data. Ten criteria for an effective MIS are the following: informative, relevant, sensitive, unbiased, comprehensive, timely, action-oriented, uniform, performance-targeted, and cost effective. A *clinical data repository* is a physical or logical compilation of client data pertaining to health.

Automated information systems are useful for collecting clinical data to direct client care and manage care processes. There have been great strides in medical data collection and analysis, but nursing lags behind in the development of support systems because of lack of consensus on how nursing knowledge is represented and on how nurses make decisions. The standardization of a nursing data set is essential to capture the contributions that nurses make to client care. Reimbursement decisions are made based on hard data that are easily retrievable and show positive outcomes. Four domains of nursing's data needs include the client data, provider data, administrative data, and research data. Nurses must clearly define their data elements, identify linkages between and among data sets, and design a clear coding system to ensure usable data sets. The determination of data elements and engineering technology are important aspects of nursing informatics.

The American Nurses Association established the Nursing Information and Data Set Evaluation Center (NIDSEC) in 1995 to assist nurses with vendor evaluation. The NIDSEC has established standards and scoring guidelines for venders wishing to be approved. Currently, nine classifications for nursing care are recognized by the American Nurses Association. The approved classifications include North American Nursing Diagnosis Association, Nursing Intervention Classification, Nursing Outcomes Classification, Nursing Management Minimum Data Set, Home Health Care Classification, OMAHA system, Patient Care Data Set, Perioperative Nursing Data Set, and Systematized Nomenclature of Human and Veterinary Medicine.

Computerized patient records are designed to provide a longitudinal account of care, an information system that tracks care in a variety of settings, and a tracking mechanism of care across settings and time. The advantages of a computerized patient record include readily available access to longitudinal records linked over time, access to real-time availability, legible records, triggers, and reminders. Barriers to the use of a computerized patient record include readiness, security, confidentiality issues, complexity, and volume of data. The development and use of computerized patient records may include systems that alert clinicians to abnormal data, contain clinical decision support systems, and link knowledge bases.

Large databases are now being developed to collect information on health care workers and client care. Examples include the Institute of Medicine's Computer-Based Patient Record of an account of client care and the American Nurses Association's Nursing Information System (NIS), which keeps records of nurses' licensure and credentials. There are many advantages to large data sets, but there are also limitations. Problems can include flawed data, inadequate methodologies, and the misuse of sensitive health care information on practitioner practice patterns.

The result of computerized applications to nursing administration for nurse leaders is the designing of an integrated management information system that uses standardized nursing language and data elements for comparative purposes. To advocate the inclusion of essential nursing data elements in national databases is crucial for nursing practice and reimbursement. The Uniform Hospital Discharge Data Set does not include nursing data elements because nursing lacks a standardized data set that is clearly defined, valid, and reliable. Nurses are challenged to identify and validate a standardized nursing data set to ensure inclusion in national data sets. Such efforts are currently underway for nursing administration. The *Nursing Management Minimum Data Set* (NMMDS) is a database that includes service-related management data elements. Data elements include cost, quality, and outcome data. The limitations of the NMMDS are that nursing practice and personnel data about individual nurses is omitted, and it lacks uniform collection practices across sites.

Nursing leadership is needed to provide innovations in data management and informatics to enhance client care. Data security and confidentiality are key components in managing information systems. A current trend in data management and informatics is the continued growth of managed care as a market force driving extensive changes in the use of information technology. It is postulated that health care in the United States will undergo a major reorganization and that large, multistate managed care plans will emerge as the primary providers of health services. The five tools as emerging technologies in nursing include the internet, continuous speech recognition, wireless computing, thin-client computing, and data warehouses (Simpson, 1999).

LEARNING TOOLS

Activity: Domains of Nursing Data

Purpose: To identify essential elements in the four domains of nursing data.

Directions: Using the following spaces for each of the four domains of nursing data listed, identify elements in each domain that would be important to collect and analyze in an NIS. Review Table 32–1 for outcomes and variables in the three domains of nursing data needs, and review Figure 32–1 for proposed NMMDS elements.

	Client	Domains Provider	Administrative
Outcomes	Client satisfaction Achieved care outcomes Costs Access to care	Job enrichment Job/work satisfaction Physician satisfaction Job stress Intent to leave	Costs Productivity Turnover Income
Variables	Attitudes/beliefs Diagnosis, gender, age Marital status Support system Satisfaction Level of dependency Severity of illness Intensity of nursing care	Attitudes/beliefs Education Years of experience Age Work excitement	Agency philosophy Priorities Organizational structure Fiscal data Climate Policies and procedures Conflict

Table 32–1. Outcomes and Variables in Three Domains of Nursing Data Needs

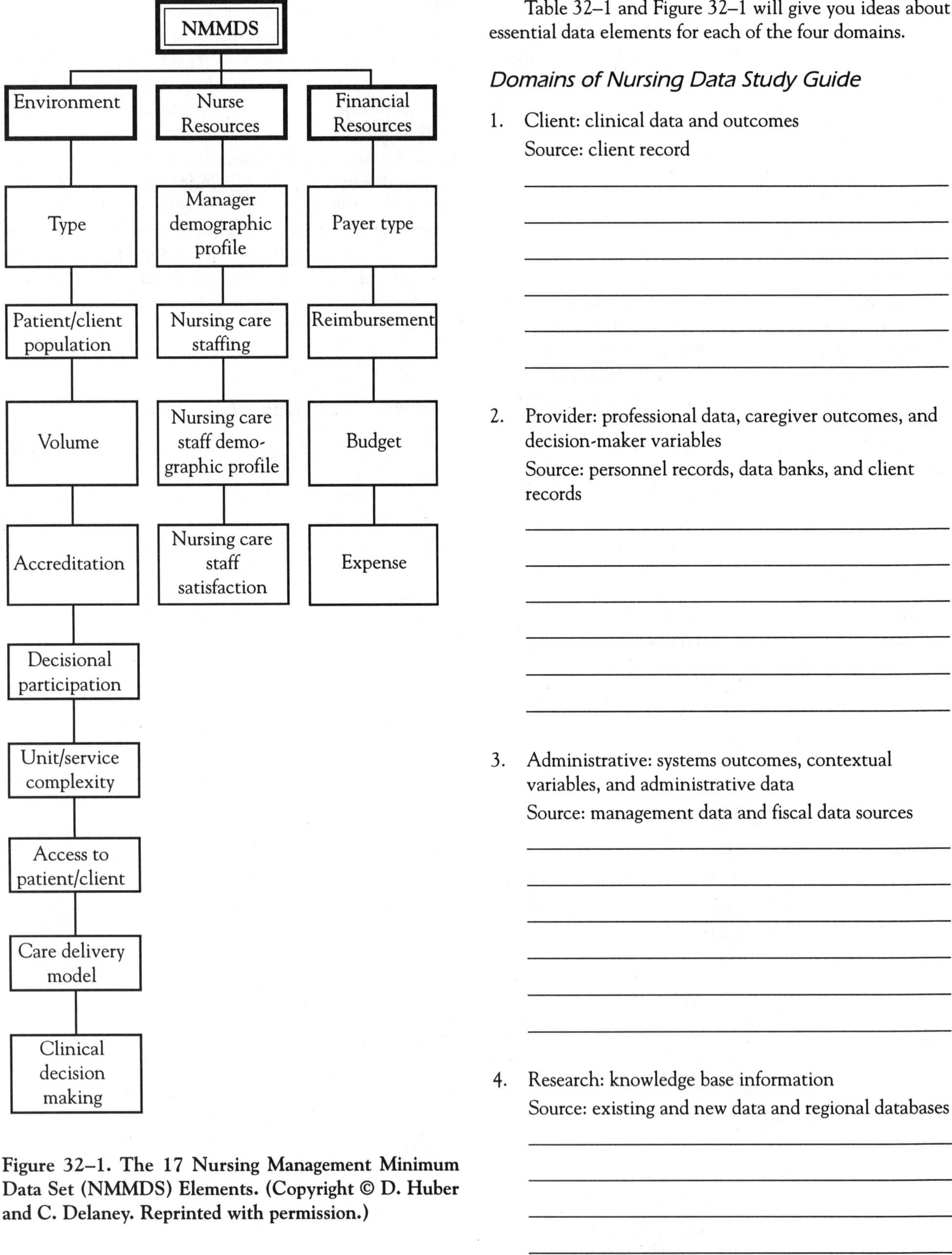

Figure 32–1. The 17 Nursing Management Minimum Data Set (NMMDS) Elements. (Copyright © D. Huber and C. Delaney. Reprinted with permission.)

Table 32–1 and Figure 32–1 will give you ideas about essential data elements for each of the four domains.

Domains of Nursing Data Study Guide

1. Client: clinical data and outcomes

   Source: client record

   ____

   ____

   ____

   ____

   ____

   ____

2. Provider: professional data, caregiver outcomes, and decision-maker variables

   Source: personnel records, data banks, and client records

   ____

   ____

   ____

   ____

   ____

   ____

3. Administrative: systems outcomes, contextual variables, and administrative data

   Source: management data and fiscal data sources

   ____

   ____

   ____

   ____

   ____

   ____

4. Research: knowledge base information

   Source: existing and new data and regional databases

   ____

   ____

   ____

   ____

   ____

   ____

Each of the four nursing domains is important to include in NIS and MIS. Identifying essential variables and outcome by nursing unit and by institution is critical in obtaining quantifiable comparable data. This data can be used to compare units within an institution, as well as across institutions. The collection and analysis of basic nursing data sets are important for nursing to demonstrate nurses' unique contribution to client care.

CASE STUDY

Jackie is a nursing director of critical care and has been asked to make recommendations for purchasing a nursing information system (NIS) for a large teaching hospital. Jackie is very knowledgeable about clinical issues, but has not had much experience with computers or information systems. Jackie reads about NIS and MIS and wonders if purchasing an MIS would not be a better choice for the organization. She struggles to determine which data elements are essential when purchasing a NIS.

Case Study Questions

1. Would an MIS meet the needs of a nurse administrator?
2. Is there an advantage to a nurse administrator in purchasing an NIS over an MIS?
3. What four domains of nursing data should Jackie remember to include as criteria for selection of an NIS?

LEARNING RESOURCES

Discussion Questions

1. What is the difference between informatics and nursing informatics?
2. What is effectiveness research and how can it be useful in nursing practice?
3. How can standardized nursing data sets help nurses gain reimbursement status for nursing services?
4. Should the NMMDS be refined or should a new data set be designed? Why?
5. Identify benefits of an NIS for clinical nurses. Identify any barriers for clinical nurses in using an NIS.

Study Questions

Matching: Write the letter of the correct response in front of each term.

_____ 1. Nursing informatics
_____ 2. Informatics
_____ 3. Computer
_____ 4. Effectiveness research
_____ 5. Management information system
_____ 6. Computer-based patient record
_____ 7. NMMDS
_____ 8. Quality improvement tools
_____ 9. Clinical data repository
_____ 10. Nursing Information and Data Set Evaluation Center

A. Tool for managing data
B. Analysis of large databases using epidemiological methods
C. Combination of computer and information science
D. Integrated system to collect and manipulate data for the purposes of directing and controlling resources
E. Management of data to support the practice and delivery of nursing care
F. Tracks longitudinal accounts of client care
G. Identifies common causes of variation and visual display of data
H. Physical or logical compilation of client data pertaining to health
I. A center that assists nurses with vendor evaluation of automated information systems or computer-based client record systems
J. Elements crucial to evaluation of nursing interventions on client outcomes

REFERENCES

Newbold, S. (1998). Information systems for managing patient care. In J.A. Dienemann (Ed.), *Nursing Administration: Managing Patient Care* (2nd ed.), pp. 323-338. Stamford, CT: Appleton & Lange.

Simpson, R.L. (1999). What does IT have in store for nursing? *Nursing Management, 30(10)*, 14-15.

SUPPLEMENTAL READINGS

Henry, S.B., Douglas, K., Galzagorry, G., Lahey, A. & Holzemer, W.L. (1998). A template-based approach to support utilization of clinical practice guidelines within an electronic health record. *Journal of the American Medical Informatics, 5(3)*, 237-244, 248.

Hughes, M. (1999). Information in resource management: Ward managers' perception, *Health Informatics Journal, 5(1)*, 20-29.

Pearson, C. & Williams, J. (1998). Learning and culture change: Towards better information management and patient care. *British Journal of Healthcare Computing & Information Management, 15(8)*, 40-43.

Simpson, R.L. (1998). Technology: Nursing the system. A NIDSEC primer: part 2—setting the standards... Nursing informatics and data set evaluation center. *Nursing Management, 29(2)*, 26-27, 29.

Tak, S.H., Nield, M. & Becker, H. (1999). Nursing informatics. Use of a computer software program for qualitative analysis—part 2: Advantages and disadvantages... NUD-IST. *Western Journal of Nursing Research, 21(3)*, 436-439.

ANSWERS TO TEXT STUDY QUESTIONS

Chapter 32—Data Management and Informatics (p. 606)

1. **What role do computers play in nursing care?**

   Computers play a vital role in facilitating nursing care. Nursing informatics is the management and processing of nursing data, information, and knowledge to support care delivery. The use of computerized technology to collect data, document, and rapidly retrieve critical information is essential in care delivery. As a nursing tool, informatics affords nursing the opportunity to collect, process, and retrieve data to support the use of resources, optimize patient outcomes and to compare data. Clinical decisions made from reliable data augments the decision-making process and supports positive patient outcomes.

2. **Who uses nursing's data?**

   Clinicians, academicians, nurse leaders, and administrators use nursing data. The data are used to guide client care decisions, determine patient census and acuity, and assist in strategic planning and quality management activities. Additionally, nursing leaders use nursing-sensitive data to demonstrate the impact and efficacy of nursing care within an organizational system.

3. **What are the data used for?**

   Data can be used to augment decisional support for the client, health care provider, and organization. Clinical data and information are used to address issues related to quality, effectiveness, and client outcomes. Regulatory bodies review nursing data to determine compliance to policies and regulations.

4. **What difference do nurses who manage health care services make? Under what circumstances?**

   Nurses who manage health care services bring to light data that demonstrate the contribution of nursing to the organization. The collection, analysis, and dissemination of data recognize and emphasize the role nursing plays in managing cost-effective health care outcomes. As such, nursing's unique role becomes visible and recognized by physician colleagues, hospital administrators, and reimbursement agencies.

5. **What are the cost, quality, and satisfaction outcomes for which nurses are mainly responsible?**

   Nursing practice impacts all cost, quality, and client satisfaction outcomes. Examples of cost outcomes include length of stay, supply cost per unit of service, and labor costs by acuity level per client. Quality outcomes include medication errors, documentation compliance, and infection rates. Satisfaction outcomes may include ratings by clients, nurses, and physicians related to client care services.

6. **Which data need to be client specific, nurse specific, and organization specific?**

   Client-specific data include clinical data related to the client, the client's plan of care, and evaluation of interventions. Nurse-specific data include licensure, certification and competencies, and employee satisfaction. Organizational-specific data elements include human and fiscal resource statistics; recruitment and retention figures; quality and effectiveness measures; and variables reflecting access, availability, and utilization of health care services.

Quality Improvement and Risk Management

STUDY FOCUS

Quality improvement is an essential component of health care and is linked with evaluation and accountability. There is tremendous pressure on health care organizations to deliver high-quality care at lower costs in order to compete successfully in a competitive environment. *Quality* is the provision of excellent care that is effective, efficient, and appropriate. *Quality of care* refers to the delivery of health care services and the belief that using up-to-date professional knowledge will likely result in positive outcomes. *Assurance* is the completion of services in an excellent manner. *Quality assurance* is the provision of services according to professional standards in a manner acceptable to the client. *Quality improvement programs* are implemented organization-wide to ensure accountability to clients and payers. *Total quality process* or *total quality management* is a method of including all employees in the improvement of services to ensure client satisfaction. *Continuous quality improvement* is a multidisciplinary process to improve systems by analyzing performance, collecting data, and changing archaic or inefficient systems. *Indicators* are valid and reliable quantitative measures of structure, process, or outcomes related to one or more dimensions of performance. *Clinical indicators* are related to clients. *Sentinel events* measure a low-volume, but serious, undesirable and potentially avoidable, process or outcome. *Benchmarking* is a tool to measure what exists against the best practices in the industry. *Best practice* is a service, function, or process that is implemented to produce superior outcomes. *Standards* are written value statements. The three basic types of standards for health care include structure, process, and outcome.

Cost, equity, access, and quality considerations underlie health care policies and decisions. Quality assessment (measurement) activities began in the 1880s with Florence Nightingale collecting data and developing standards. Quality assessment has evolved from close scrutiny and the monitoring of quality indicators (quality assurance) to the system-wide implementation of multidisciplinary teams in a continuous effort to improve systems (total quality improvement). Trends in quality improvement include the development of interdisciplinary quality assurance teams, client satisfaction, quality circles and councils, and the automation of quality indicators.

W. Edward Deming was influential in alerting Americans to the necessity of commitment to quality and listening to the customer's concerns. He used a unit-based approach focused on using higher quality to entice loyal customers. Key principles necessary for continuous quality improvement include organizational commitment, an understanding of individual client needs, continuously improving process, commitment to high-quality services, use of data, commitment by top management, benchmarking, and the formation of long-term relationships with a few suppliers.

Regulatory agencies impact organizational standards and quality by establishing minimal levels for compliance. The Joint Commission on Accreditation of Healthcare Organizations (JCAHO) accredits health care organizations in ambulatory care, long-term care, psychiatric care, home care, and hospitals. JCAHO is a private, not-for-profit organization that was founded in 1951. Without accreditation, Medicare and Medicaid reimbursement will not be paid to a health care agency. The JCAHO ten-step process for quality assurance includes assigning responsibility, delineating the scope of practice, identifying important aspects of care, designating specific indicators of care, establishing thresholds for evaluation, collecting data, evaluating care, acting to solve problems, assessing actions and documenting improvement, and communicating quality. By the end of the 1990s, JCAHO had moved into its ORYX initiative, which integrates the use of outcomes and other performance measures into the accreditation process. Part of the initiative is aimed at identifying a core set of evidence-based and soundly tested performance measures.

Standards are established by professional organizations and regulatory agencies and can be written in terms of structure, process, or outcomes. Professional organizations are the authoritative source for professional standards of practice. Standards define quality from which outcomes and performance can be measured. *Structural standards* focus on the internal organization and its personnel. *Process standards* measure activities, and outcome standards measure whether the services made a difference. A *standard of care* is outcome-oriented and identifies what the client can expect. A standard of practice is process-oriented and identifies what the provider must do to achieve the standard of care.

Standards are measured by audits, which may be concurrent or retrospective. Concurrent audits are ongoing while the client is receiving services; whereas retrospective audits occur after the services are provided. Documentation is the core source of audits. Statistical tools, histograms, control charts, scatter diagrams, run charts, and pareto charts manipulate data expressed in numbers and describe quantitative data. Nonstatistical tools, process flow diagrams, fishbone diagrams, or cause-and-effect diagrams describe qualitative data and can be expressed visually. Research and quality assessment are both evaluation techniques. Research is highly controlled and experimental. Quality assessment is day-to-day evaluation. Research is intended to be generalizable, but quality assurance is to determine effectiveness, efficiency, and appropriateness of care. Quality assurance evaluation tends to identify researchable problems, while research can strengthen a quality improvement program.

Professions monitor their own practice to set standards and ensure public accountability. Many professions require ongoing continuing education as a mechanism to ensure that their members stay current. Risk management programs are organizational methods of identifying risks, controlling occurrences, preventing damage, and controlling legal liability. The goal of risk management departments is to minimize financial loss due to malpractice claims. Risk management activities are focused on high-risk behaviors or areas in an attempt to prevent accidents. Organizations typically use incident reports to determine high-risk activities, track them, and implement control programs to prevent further occurrences.

LEARNING TOOLS

Activity: Organizational Quality Improvement Assessment

Purpose: To assess the level of continuous quality improvement in the organization in which you work.

Directions: Read each statement below, and then circle the number that best describes your assessment.

Key: 1–not at all, 2–to a small extent, 3–to a moderate extent, 4–to a great extent, and 5–to a very great extent

1. Employees clearly understand who the customer is. 1 2 3 4 5
2. All employees clearly understand the customer's needs. 1 2 3 4 5
3. There is regular contact with the customer. 1 2 3 4 5
3. There is ongoing quality assessment of the customer's needs and what is actually provided. 1 2 3 4 5
5. Employees work in interdisciplinary teams. 1 2 3 4 5
6. Employees independently identify problems and seek to improve them. 1 2 3 4 5
7. Employees handle customer complaints autonomously. 1 2 3 4 5
8. Employees are valued and treated with respect. 1 2 3 4 5
9. Employees are allowed to do what it takes to do a high-quality job. 1 2 3 4 5
10. Employees are encouraged to handle work problems. 1 2 3 4 5
11. Employees do not need managerial approval to handle problems. 1 2 3 4 5

12. Experimentation and risk taking is valued and encouraged. 1 2 3 4 5

13. Change is viewed positively by employees. 1 2 3 4 5

14. Employees are encouraged to meet and discuss work. 1 2 3 4 5

15. Employees feel free to discuss matters openly and have no fear about disagreeing or offering alternative solutions. 1 2 3 4 5

16. Failures are viewed as learning opportunities and are not punished. 1 2 3 4 5

17. Managers facilitate employees' work and encourage input into work activities and consumer needs. 1 2 3 4 5

18. Communication is open, and employees are kept informed of changes. 1 2 3 4 5

19. Group members work cohesively and share recognition for team accomplishments. 1 2 3 4 5

20. Individuals in top management positions are visible and encourage employee input into organizational matters. 1 2 3 4 5

21. Employees enjoy and have fun at work. 1 2 3 4 5

21. Innovation is encouraged, facilitated, and supported. 1 2 3 4 5

Scoring: Add up the total score for all 22 items. The higher the score the more apt your organization is to have a quality improvement program or strong elements of a program in place. Organizations that have continuous quality improvement programs tend to value employees, satisfy customers, and continually improve the process and services provided. Innovations are prized and risk taking is encouraged.

CASE STUDY

Pat is a master's-prepared nurse who has been asked by the chief executive officer (CEO) of a medium-sized community hospital in Waterloo, Tennessee, to develop an organization-wide program to monitor major occurrences. Pat knows that there is an incident report system currently in place at the hospital, but the only people who see the reports are the managers. Pat decides to centralize the incident report system, identify and track major occurrences, and develop programs to minimize incidents. Pat decides to create a task force composed of employees and managers to relate her concerns and to elicit feedback. The CEO has informed Pat that one of her responsibilities is to decrease the amount and number of malpractice claims.

Case Study Questions

1. What type of program is Pat designing?
2. Is the program Pat is designing a component of quality improvement?
3. Should incident reports be used in a punitive manner?

LEARNING RESOURCES

Discussion Questions

1. Describe what continuous quality improvement (CQI) is, and identify key elements of a CQI program.
2. What are the similarities and differences in quality assessment and research?
3. What is the ten-step process of quality assurance for organizations as outlined by JCAHO?
4. Why do health care organizations seek accreditation from JCAHO?
5. What is the difference between a standard of care and a standard of practice?
6. What is the difference between research and quality assurance?

Study Questions

True or False: Circle the correct answer.

T F 1. A standard of care is outcome-oriented and focuses on the nurse as a provider.

T F 2. The three areas in which quality can be measured are structure, process, and cost.

T F 3. A feature of a profession is that it monitors its own practice.

T F 4. Risk management programs are designed to assure a high level of quality.

T F 5. Once an incident report is filled out, it absolves the person from responsibility for the occurrence.

T F 6. Standards can only be set by professional organizations.

T F 7. Retrospective audits are popular because an organization can monitor the client's progress while he or she is receiving services.

T F 8. Today, emphasis is on outcomes rather than process.

T F 9. Continuous quality improvement aims to develop long-term relationships with a few suppliers and is responsive to customer needs.

T F 10. Quality assurance is a highly controlled experimental research of client services.

T F 11. Medicare and Medicaid reimbursement will not be paid to health care organizations that are not accredited.

T F 12. JCAHO founded in 1951, is a private, not-for-profit organization that is an accrediting body for hospitals and health care organizations.

SUPPLEMENTAL READINGS

Johnson, C.G. (1999). "Knock-your-socks-off" service. *Nursing Management, 30(7)*, 16-19.

Koivula, M., Paunonen, M., & Laippala, P. (1998). Prerequisites for quality improvement in nursing. *Journal of Nursing Management*, *6(6)*, 332-342.

ANSWERS TO TEXT STUDY QUESTIONS

Chapter 33—Quality Improvement and Risk Management (p. 630)

1. **Who is responsible for quality management?**

   Quality management is the responsibility of the organization and the providers. All levels of management and care providers are accountable for the knowledge of and adherence to standards of care. The professional nurse is responsible for monitoring her or his own practice relative to improving care delivery.

2. **What are the differences between institutional and professional responsibilities for quality? Why does this occur?**

   Institutional responsibilities for quality are directly linked to organizational efforts to provide a quality health care system. These responsibilities often include meeting external mandates for accreditation and reimbursement requirements. The professional responsibility for quality is more directly related to practice issues, client outcomes, and standards of care.

3. **How is quality defined? How is it measured?**

   Quality is defined as the characteristics manifested in the pursuit of excellence. It has been defined in terms of effectiveness and efficiency, benefits and harms, or appropriateness of care. Quality exists when outcomes compare favorably with standards and is measured by evaluating structure, process, and outcomes; relating outcomes to standards; and measuring performance. Structure focuses on the internal characteristics of an organization and its personnel; process examines the activities and interventions used to attain outcomes; and outcomes are measured by evaluating the services.

4. **How is the implementation of total quality management/continuous quality improvement affected by outcomes management?**

   Outcomes management has affected the implementation of total quality management and continuous quality improvement strategies by changing the emphasis from the assurance of quality to the measurement of quality. Concurrently, a paradigm shift occurred that changed the focus from being provider-based to one with a customer-based perspective. As such, new indicators of quality, such as adherence to professional practice standards and customer satisfaction were developed to demonstrate the excellence and efficiency of the care delivered.

5. **What components of continuous quality improvements are easiest/hardest to implement? Why?**

   The easiest components of continuous quality improvement to implement are identifying key processes in the organization in need of improvement, designating multidisciplinary teams, and scheduling meetings. The hardest continuous quality improvements to implement are shifting from a provider focus to a customer focus, eliciting active participation of all employees in the continuous improvement process, and changing managerial performance expectations.

6. **How are research and quality management related? Can they be combined in one program?**

   Both research and quality management focus on problem identification, measurement, resolution, and change. The focus of research is to generate knowledge that will inform clinical practice and improve client outcomes. In comparison, the focus of quality management is on excellence, adherence to performance standards, and the reduction of waste and costs. Incorporating research into quality management strengthens performance measures and the evaluation of care standards.

7. **What is the relationship of payment to level of quality?**

   Maintaining a minimum level of quality in care delivery is mandated by accreditation agencies. Without accreditation, reimbursement from federal agencies can be jeopardized or withheld. Medicare and Medicaid programs will not reimburse health care organizations without current JCAHO accreditation.

Strategic Management

STUDY FOCUS

Strategic planning is important in health care to find ways to gain a competitive edge in a highly competitive environment. *Strategic planning* is a systematic process of making entrepreneurial decisions, planning for implementation, and evaluating outcomes (Drucker, 1974). *Strategic management* is a broad concept that includes strategic planning and focuses on important aspects of strategy implementation. Strategic management assists nurses in responding to turbulent changes and capturing opportunities that increase the likelihood of achieving desired outcomes.

A *strategy* is a broad, integrated plan of action aimed at accomplishing organizational goals (Hersey, Blanchard, & Johnson, 1996). A *tactic* is a device used to implement a strategy (Nierenburg, 1995). Strategy comes first and then tactics follow. Tactics are quick, specialized, flexible, less predictable, more glorious, and dangerous (Beckham, 1990). Examples of tactics include boldness, simplicity, surprise, deception, and intimidation (Beckham, 1990). A *strategic plan* is a written document for allocating resources to accomplish organizational goals. *Organizational effectiveness* is performing similar activities better than rivals do. Strategic positioning is performing different activities from what rivals do. *Opportunistic planning* is aimed at tactics and day-to-day operations with constant improvement a key feature; whereas, strategic planning reflects the organizations response to key issues and future goals. A reliance on constant improvement and best practices alone may result in imitation and homogeneity (Potter, 1996). Strategic positions need to be a decade or longer to ensure continuity and reinforce the identity of the organization.

Traditional planning relies on historical data projected into the future. In rapidly changing environments, proactive, flexible, and creative strategic plans are vital to success. Strategic plans force tough choices in resource allocation and attempt to align organizational capabilities with external opportunities. The two distinct phases of the strategic management process are development and implementation of strategy (Maljers, 1990). Anticipating and managing surprise is an important aspect of organizational management. The three phases of the strategic management process include developing an environmental analysis, designing a strategic plan, and establishing a time line. An internal and external organizational analysis is critical in the strategic management process. External analysis includes strengths, weaknesses, opportunities, and threats (SWOT). The key principle is that systematic and careful analysis of environmental factors and trends increase the likelihood that the impact of change will be accurately gauged and proactive organizational direction will occur. Questions organizations must tackle include: What might we do? What can we do? What do we want to do? and What should we do?

The strategic planning process should include everyone in the organization (Peters, 1987). The eight phases of the strategic planning process are beginning, preparing, analyzing information, ends planning, means planning, controlling, completing a written strategic plan, and implementing the plan. The important functions of strategic planning are analyzing the environment by considering opportunities, establishing measurable organizational goals, and creating the organization's mission and purpose. Central to planning is the continuous research about the organization and the environment. Questions that form the basis of strategic planning are related to the business of nursing, the discipline of nursing, the goals, market forces, strategy, and management of change. The elements of a strategic plan include an executive summary, introduction and background, description of the strategic plan, internal and external assessment, description of the structure and management, program requirements, marketing, and financial and implementation plan.

Strategic management is a leadership tool designed to provide competitive advantage for organizations. The strategic planning process creates a spirit of partnership and cooperation among internal and external organizational players. The results of planning may increase ownership, improve morale, and increase commitment by all stakeholders. Strategic plans need to be realistic and future-oriented.

Intrapreneurs are individuals in an organization who design new products or services. *Entrepreneurs* are individuals who establish their own businesses. An entrepreneurial opportunity must be a desirable future state involving change or growth and the individual must believe that he or she can reach the goal (Stevenson & Gumpert, 1992). Business and marketing plans are essential elements of a strategic plan. In organizations, a feasibility study is often used, as it is a modified business plan developed to capture internal resources. For those who plan to establish their own company, a business plan is essential. A business plan is a written document that summarizes the business opportunity and specifies the plan for capitalizing on the opportunity.

LEARNING TOOLS

Case Study

Sam is a staff nurse who is employed by a large teaching hospital in Phoenix, Arizona. She works the 3-11 shift on a 65-bed medical-surgical unit. Sam is very creative and enjoys patient education. She makes sure that every client that she cares for begins educational activities the day they are admitted to ensure mastery of material prior to discharge. Sam has designed a novel approach to patient education for individuals who undergo a hysterectomy. She has designed a game for them to play, which provides postoperative care and instructions for home care. The patients all comment on how useful the game is and how much they enjoy this approach to learning. Sam's peers are requesting that she provide the games for other units and she is receiving requests from nurses employed at other hospitals to use the games that she has designed. Sam decides that she would like to expand this concept and make the patient education games available to other hospitals.

Case Study Questions

1. Who should Sam approach to gain support for further development of the teaching tool?
2. Is Sam an intrapreneur or an entrepreneur?
3. Should a feasibility study or a business plan be developed?
4. What types of intrapreneurial and entrepreneurial activities can nurses engage?

LEARNING RESOURCES

Group Activity: Developing a Business Plan

Introduction: Nurses are becoming more entrepreneurial and establishing businesses in communities. To be successful in developing a business it is useful to complete a business plan to develop strategies to successfully compete in the marketplace.

Directions: The group should decide upon a health care product or service that they would like to develop into a business. Once the core health care business is identified, complete the Basic Elements of a Business Plan.

Basic Elements of a Business Plan

1. Executive Summary—Provide an overview of the business, market, and profitability of the company.
2. Company Description—Provide a detailed description of the business.
3. Industry Survey—Provide a description of the history, the present state, and the future demand for the product or service.
4. Market Research—Conduct or find information that provides data regarding the product or services that is proposed.
5. Management Team—Identify the individuals who will compose the management team and identify the strengths that they bring to the company.
6. Professional Assistance—Identify the types of assistance (and names of individuals) that will be needed to form the company. For example, will attorneys, technical individuals, or accountants be needed?
7. Operational Plan—What is the time line and steps to develop the product or service. Who is accountable for each step? Are there checkpoints?
8. Research and Development—What are the plans for continued research and development? Who will be in charge of this component of the business?
9. Overall Schedule—Where is the master schedule kept and who is responsible to keep activities on schedule?
10. Risks and Opportunities—What are the risks and opportunities that the company faces today and what are potential risks and opportunities in the future?
11. Three-Year Financial Forecast—A written document that contains a three-year financial forecast should be in place and evaluation points should be identified.

12. Proposed Financing—Where will the proposed financing come? What are the plans for repayment of debt?
13. Legal Structure—How will the business be formed? Will it be a corporation?
14. Marketing Plans and Research—What are the marketing plans and strategies? What markets are targeted? What type of ongoing marketing efforts will be implemented?
15. Venture Capital—What is the financial support for the development of the product or service? Are there any grants to assist with start-up costs? Is there any community support?

Summary: A business plan is an important aspect of developing a new venture. Often a business plan is used to acquire financing, to provide strategic policy, and to attract key individuals with specialized expertise to the new organization. A well-written business plan provides strong data to determine the viability of the proposed business venture and provides a guide for measuring attainment of goals.

Discussion Questions

1. Discuss intrapreneur and entrepreneur activities that nurses in your community have designed. In a small group setting, discuss ideas and activities that could be undertaken by nurses to develop a company or enhance an organization's viability.
2. What is the relationship between strategic planning and strategic management?
3. Describe the strategic planning process.
4. What are the elements of a strategic plan?
5. What are the common features of strategic management?

Study Questions

True or False. Circle the correct answer.

T F 1. A strategy is a device used to implement actions.

T F 2. Forecasting is one technique used in strategic planning.

T F 3. Operational effectiveness is performing similar activities better than rivals do.

T F 4. Reliance on constant improvement and best practices alone moves organizations toward imitation and homogeneity.

T F 5. Strategic positions should have a horizon of no more than five years.

T F 6. There are two stages to the strategic management process: development and implementation of strategy.

T F 7. The best strategic planning is "top-down."

T F 8. The strategic planning process is very threatening to employees and creates decreased job satisfaction.

T F 9. Intrapreneurs are employees who create new programs or ventures for the organization.

T F 10. A close relationship exists between opportunity and individual need.

REFERENCES

Beckham, J.D. (1990). Tactics—The hot and sweaty work. *Healthcare Forum Journal, 33(1)*, 20-24.

Drucker, P.F. (1974). *Management: Tasks, Responsibilities, Practices*. New York: Harper & Row.

Hersey, P., Blanchard, K.H. & Johnson, D.E. (1996). *Management of Organizational Behavior: Utilizing Human Resources* (7th ed.). Upper Saddle River, NJ: Prentice-Hall.

Johnson, L. (1992). Strategic management in nursing administration. In P.J. Decker & E.J. Sullivan (Eds.), *Nursing Administration: A Micro/Macro Approach for Effective Nurse Executives* (pp. 71-100). Norwalk, CT: Appleton & Lange.

Maljers, F.A. (1990). Strategic planning and intuition in Unilever. *Long Range Planning, 23(2)*, 155-160.

Nierenberg, G.I. (1995). *The Art of Negotiating*. New York: Barnes & Noble Books.

Peters, T. (1987). *Thriving on Chaos*. New York: Harper-Collins.

Porter, M.E. (1996). What is strategy? *Harvard Business Review, 74(6)*, 61-78.

Stevenson, H.H. & Gumpert, D.E. (1992). The heart of entrepreneurship. In W.A. Sahlman, & H.H. Stevenson (Eds.), *The Entrepreneurial Venture* (pp. 9-25). Boston: Harvard Business School Publications.

SUPPLEMENTAL READINGS

Daniels, K. (1999). Affect and strategic decision making. *Psychologist, 12(1)*, 24-28.

Hoskisson, R.E., Hitt, M.A., Wan-William, P. & Yiu, D. (1999). Theory and research in strategic management: Swings of a pendulum. *Journal of Management, 25(3)*, 417-456.

Stone, M.M., Bigelow, B. & Crittenden, W. (1999). Research on strategic management in nonprofit organizations: Synthesis, analysis, and future directions. *Administration & Society, 31(3)*, 378-423.

Sullivan, M.A. & Parisi, R.A. (1999). Strategic decision making on shifting sands. *Nursing Administration Quarterly, 23(4)*, 75-80.

ANSWERS TO TEXT STUDY QUESTIONS

Chapter 34—Strategic Management (p. 640)

1. **What is strategic management? How does it differ from planning? From strategic planning?**

   Strategic management is a process concerned with fundamental organizational renewal and growth. It is a future-oriented plan that defines the trajectory of the organization's direction over a finite period of time. Strategic management differs from planning in that it is systematic, deliberate, and proactive, environmentally oriented, administrative in nature, and sensitive to the position of the organization in the community. Planning is often dependent on continuity, stability, and trend data to predict future changes and opportunities, yet it may not be long-range or responsive in nature. With this myopic perspective, organizational viability may be jeopardized. Strategic planning differs from traditional planning in that it involves the development of a detailed program of prioritized actions that will facilitate the achievement of organization's mission, vision, and goals.

2. **Why has strategic planning become important in health care settings?**

   As the health care environment has become increasingly competitive and turbulent, strategic planning is a crucial process for organizational survival. In order for organizations to exist in this type of climate, they must be willing to develop a visionary strategic plan that will facilitate service delivery, while maintaining financial viability. Strategic planning incorporates marketing strategies and initiatives that will assist in the realization of the organization's mission and provides opportunities for improvement and growth.

3. **What does a strategic plan look like?**

   A strategic plan is a written document that outlines the long-range plan for the organization. This comprehensive plan includes ten elements: (1) an executive summary; (2) an introduction and background; (3) a detailed description of the strategic plan; (4) an external assessment of the marker; (5) an internal assessment of strengths, weaknesses, opportunities, and threats; (6) a description of structure, including managerial; (7) the program requirements; (8) a marketing plan; (9) a financial plan; and (10) an implementation plan.

4. **What process is used to develop a strategic plan?**

   Johnson (1992) recommended an eight-phase process to develop a strategic plan. These phases are the beginning, preparation, information analysis, ends planning, means planning, controls, completing the written strategic plan, and implementing the strategic plan. The beginning phase reviews the mission, objectives, goals, assumptions, history, and values. In the preparation phase, the strategic plan is designed and organized. The analytic phase assesses the internal and external environment, while the ends planning phase is involved with developing and revising the mission, objectives, and goals, as well as developing future strategies. The means planning phase involves the development and initiation of strategic planning activities, while the controls phase is concerned with the development of outcomes and evaluation criteria. The final two phases of the strategic planning process involves completing the written document and implementing the strategic plan.

5. **Who should develop nursing's strategic plan? The tactics used?**

   Nurses at all levels within the organization should be involved in the development of nursing's strategic plan. Participation and input help shape the organizational assessment and create solidarity. It is crucial that those nurses who will be actualizing the strategy and those nurses who decide resource allocation be involved in its inception, development, and execution. Nurses with tactical experience can offer a variety of approaches to implement the strategic plan. Using judgment and ethical decision-making strategies, both nurse managers and nurse clinicians should collaborate to develop the most effective tactics that should be employed to realize the goals of the strategic plan.

Marketing

STUDY FOCUS

Marketing is a concept from business administration that pertains to sales, persuasion, and image projection. *Marketing* is concerned with stimulating and meeting consumer demand. The key to successful marketing is to stimulate and satisfy buyer wants and needs. Marketing is one aspect of strategic organizational planning. For-profit businesses have used marketing as a tool for many years, and not-for-profit health care organizations now use marketing in a highly competitive, resource-constrained environment to capture and maintain market share. Kotler (1999) suggests that marketing is the art of finding, developing, and profiting from opportunities.

Some individuals feel that marketing is a negative aspect in the health care environment. They feel that marketing is a waste of scarce resources, it relies on high-pressure sales, stimulating competition, creating unnecessary demand, and promoting low-quality products. However, marketing is an imperative for organizational survival in a turbulent health care environment. The three major benefits of marketing include increased client satisfaction, improved acquisition of resources, and improved organizational efficiency (Kotler & Clarke, 1987). Marketing has helped organizations cope, grow, and thrive.

A *market* is actual or potential buyers and users of goods, services, and ideas. Marketing is a social and managerial process whereby individuals or groups obtain what they need and want by a process of exchange with others. *Exchange* is the act of obtaining a valued product from someone by giving something in return (Kotler, 1988). A *marketing mix* is a blend of marketing strategies used to achieve established goals. A *marketing orientation* is focusing energy on identification of needs and on the delivery of services that create satisfied customers. Marketing orientation is also noted as customer- or consumer-focused. Market share is the percentage of the total market for the product or service that is captured by the organization. *Needs* are basic biological, psychological, and social needs. *Wants* are desires satisfied by specific products or services that are influenced by external cues. *Products* are goods, services, or ideas that satisfy wants and needs of individuals.

Markets vary depending on the geographical location, customer orientation, and service or products produced. For nurses, the primary markets are clients, the employing organization, and physicians. For health care organizations, the primary markets are clients, employees, and physicians. Marketing occurs within the context of voluntary exchange. Transactions are basic units of exchange. Values are benefits derived from the exchange minus the cost associated with the product or service. A marketing orientation is the identification of customers' needs and wants and delivering satisfactory goods in exchange for a price. Five attributes of a marketing orientation include a customer-oriented philosophy, integrated marketing organization, adequate marketing-information, strategic orientation, and operational efficiency.

The key elements of marketing are strategy and research. Four strategic planning decisions contribute to the development of a cohesive marketing plan. The four strategic decisions include defining the business, determining the mission, formulating functional strategies, and budgeting. Marketing efforts use research tools to provide a report of the opportunities and threats, market analysis, and competitor position. Market strategies may be broad or narrow. Mass marketing aims the product to the entire market, target marketing aims the product to a specific segment of the population, and customer-level marketing aims the product or services to the individual customer (Kotler, 1999). Marketing strategies are often aimed at fulfilling needs. Responsive marketing is designed to find and fill needs, anticipative marketing is designed to recognize an emerging or latent need, and need-shaped marketing is designed to introduce a new product or service.

The five steps of effective marketing are researching to uncover opportunities and data, identifying segments to target, establishing the marketing mix, implementing the marketing plan, and controlling for effectiveness. The marketing mix can be viewed from both the seller's and customer's point of view. The seller's point of view includes the four Ps of product, price, place, and promotion. The customer's point of view includes customer value, costs, convenience, and communication. The product is the core of the business and is usually an object, service, or idea. A core product is what clients seek to meet basic needs, a tangible product has characteristics of style, quality, and brand name, and augmented products have added services and benefits (Alward & Camunas, 1991; Kotler, 1999).

Services are provided in a way that the other party does not become an owner of the product. Services are differentiated from products by five characteristics: intangibility, inseparability, variability, perishability, and consumer involvement. Nurses and nursing need to capitalize on the uniqueness of the services provided. Clear articulation of the services of nurses will enhance the message and improve desired outcomes in health care. Nurses must position themselves strategically in the market by capitalizing on the five Ps of service business marketing. The five Ps include positioning by communicating nursing services, packaging to present services, promoting the products to capture more business, persuading others to buy the service, and performing high-quality care to generate more business. Pricing is an important strategy to market and sell products. Cost-based pricing adds a profit to the price of the item, whereas value-based pricing is based on the estimated value that the customer receives resulting in different pricing for different targets.

Today's health care environment is competitive, turbulent, and constantly changing. Consumers' expectations are high and they are more sophisticated and price sensitive than ever before. Consumers expect quick and convenient service delivery, high-quality products and services, and enhanced value. Brand loyalty is eroding, resulting in greater competition for consumer demand. Astute marketing strategies are based on customer value. Marketing strategies that are customer-oriented tend to focus on understanding customer needs, developing customer relationships, and learning how to keep and grow customers (Kotler, 1999). Critical to the success of health care organizations is the development of a marketing orientation. Nursing leaders need to develop an attractive product to market to consumer groups.

Ethical issues may arise around marketing of health care products and services. There are issues surrounding price and profit in selling health care services and protecting the public. There are ethical questions around issues such as end-of-life care, organ procurement, human genome therapy, and health care as a right/cost. Nurses and nurse leaders will struggle with ethical issues in health care and provide leadership in ethical decision making.

Leadership is needed in nursing to gain a competitive advantage in marketing nursing products and services to consumer groups. Strategies to cope with the rapidly changing health care environment include analyzing the business through five categories: outputs, personnel, resources, operations, and customers (Zell, 1999). Gathering and analyzing information is imperative to competing in the health care environment. A strong customer service orientation is a key to gaining and maintaining market share. Nursing must also step forward and take leadership positions in the health care market. Seven sources of innovative opportunity include the unexpected, the incongruent, innovation based on process need, change in industry or market structure, demographic change, change in perception, mood, and meaning, and new knowledge (Drucker, 1985).

LEARNING TOOLS

Case Study

Shawmee has recently been hired as the vice president of nursing for a large health care center in Pensacola, Florida. Shawmee is impressed with the quality of health care services provided in the inpatient and outpatient areas. She notes extensive interdisciplinary team building, consultation, and sharing of key information throughout the organization. Clients who receive care at the community hospital rate the services as exceptional. Shawmee reviews trend data for both inpatient and outpatient nursing services and notes a flat line trend. There is neither growth nor retrenchment in service utilization. Shawmee feels that with the outstanding health care services provided by the employees of the community health care center that there should be a steady growth in utilization. She bases this assumption on the fact that the population in the five-county region is growing at approximately 6% annually. Shawmee contacts the media relations department for the health center and inquires about the marketing plan and strategies for the organization. The director of media relations informs Shawmee that there is not an active marketing campaign as the number of visits to the facility has been stable and there has been no need to spend money on marketing. Shawmee notes that the other health care organizations in their market area use a multitude of marketing strategies such as advertising in the newspaper, on the radio and television, providing community activities and workshops, and doing large mailings to alert consumers of new services that are being provided. Shawmee schedules an appointment with the chief executive officer to discuss marketing for the community health care center.

Case Study Questions

1. Is marketing effort necessary at the community health center? Provide rationale for your answer.
2. What are the steps in effective marketing?
3. What are the ethical implications for marketing health care services? What is the role of nurses in ethical decision making?
4. What are the major attributes of a marketing orientation?
5. Who in an organization should be responsible for marketing? Is there a role for nurses in marketing?
6. Should nurses market their services to the community? Provide a rationale for your answer.

LEARNING RESOURCES

Group Activity

Purpose: To identify a potential health care product or service that could be packaged and marketed to the community. To identify the essential elements of a marketing plan and to evaluate marketing strategies for the new health care product or service.

Directions: Identify the health care product or service that you feel has business potential. Then, complete the Marketing Study Guide to help determine what work would need to be done to develop, market, and sell the product or services.

Marketing Study Guide

Section One: Four Strategic Planning Decisions that Contribute to the Development of a Cohesive Marketing Plan

1. What is the core business?
____
2. What is the mission?
____
3. What is the marketing strategy?
____
4. What budget is needed?
____

Section Two: Attributes of a Marketing Orientation

1. Is there a customer-oriented philosophy?
____
2. Is there an integrated marketing organization?
____
3. Is their adequate marketing information?
____
4. Is there a strategic orientation?
____
5. Is there operational efficiency?
____

Section Three: Marketing Process

1. Has research been undertaken to uncover opportunities and provide data for strategic planning?
____
2. Have the segments to target been determined? If so, what are they?
____
3. What is the optimal tactical marketing mix?
____
4. Has the marketing plan been implemented with specific time lines and authority checkpoints?
____
5. What is the plan for evaluating the effectiveness of the marketing strategies and has it been implemented?
____

Section Four: Five Ps of Service Business Marketing

1. Has the message of why nursing is a valuable business partner, product, or service been communicated? What is the message?
____
2. What is the packaging to present the product or service and to generate interest?
____
3. What are the promotion strategies to maintain and acquire more business?
____
4. What persuasion strategies are being developed and implemented to sell the service or product?
____
5. What is the performance that will generate repeat business and new customers?
____

Section Five: Strategies Based on Customer Value

1. What are the customer's needs?
____
2. Have customer relationships been established?
____
3. What are the strategies to keep and grow customers?
____

Section Six: Change

1. Are systems in place to cope and develop a competitive advantage as change occurs?
____

2. What are the outputs, personnel, resources, and operations that are needed to change?

 ____

3. How will the change affect customers?

 ____

4. What marketing strategies will be needed to make a successful change?

 ____

Summary: This exercise is to assist individuals to explore entrepreneurial ideas and to determine what steps need to be taken to develop a business. There are many opportunities for nurses to develop products or services in health care to meet client needs. Historically, nurses have been hesitant to establish businesses and compete in the health care market. Today, nurses are stepping forward to design products and services that are unique to nursing and satisfy consumer needs.

Discussion Questions

1. What strategic planning decisions contribute to the development of a cohesive marketing plan?
2. What is a core product, tangible product, and augmented product?
3. What is the marketing mix from the seller's point of view and from the customer's point of view?
4. What are responsive marketing, anticipative marketing, and need-shaped marketing?
5. What are the five Ps of service business marketing?

Study Questions

Matching. Write the letter of the correct response in front of each term.

_____ 1. Market
_____ 2. Marketing
_____ 3. Exchange
_____ 4. Marketing mix
_____ 5. Marketing orientation
_____ 6. Market share
_____ 7. Needs
_____ 8. Wants
_____ 9. Products

A. A blend of marketing strategies used to achieve established goals
B. The percentage of the total market for the product or service that is captured by the organization
C. Goods, services, or ideas that satisfy wants and needs of individuals
D. Actual or potential buyers and users of goods, services, and ideas
E. Desires satisfied by specific products or services that are influenced by external cues
F. Focusing energy on identification of needs and on the delivery of services that create satisfied customers
G. Basic biological, psychological, and social needs
H. The act of obtaining a valued product from someone by giving something in return
I. A social and managerial process whereby individuals or groups obtain what they need and want by a process of exchange with others

True or False: Circle the correct answer.

T F 1. Marketing is a process that relates to transactions in an exchange of goods and services in a market.

T F 2. Marketing is only used in for-profit businesses as a strategy to increase market share.

T F 3. Marketing occurs within a framework of voluntary exchange.

T F 4. Target marketing offers a product to the entire market.

T F 5. Anticipative marketing is designed to find and fill needs.

REFERENCES

Alward, R.R. & Camunas, C. (1991). *The Nurse's Guide to Marketing.* Albany, NY: Delmar Publishers.

Drucker, P.F. (1985). *Innovations and Entrepreneurship: Practice and Principles.* New York: Harper & Row.

Kotler, P. (1988). *Marketing Management: Analysis, Planning, Implementation, and Control* (6th ed.). Englewood Cliffs, NJ: Prentice-Hall.

Kotler, P. (1999). *Kotler on Marketing: How to Create, Win, and Dominate Markets.* New York: The Free Press.

Kotler, P. & Clarke, R.N. (1987). *Marketing for Health Care Organizations.* Englewood Cliffs, NJ: Prentice Hall.

Zell, A.J. (1999). *Change—An Opportunity. {On-line}.* Available: http://www.marketingsource.com/articles/local/changeopportunity.htm.

SUPPLEMENTAL READINGS

Aydlotte, J.H. (1998). From nurse to marketing entrepreneur. *Seminars for Nurse Managers, 6(1)*, 26-29.

Kingman, M. (1998). Marketing and nursing in a competitive environment. *International Nursing Review, 45(2)*, 45-50.

Procter, S.R. & Wright, G.H. (1998). Can services marketing concepts be applied to health care? *Journal of Nursing Management, 6(3)*, 147-153.

Roberts, P.M. (1998). Nurse education in competitive markets: The case for relationship marketing. *Nurse Education Today, 18(7)*, 542-552.

Schmidt, D.Y. (1999). Financial and operational skills for nurse managers. *Nursing Administration Quarterly, 23(4)*, 16-28.

Waxman, K.T. (1998). Marketing your skills outside the hospital walls. *Nursing Management, 29(8)*, 48-52.

ANSWERS TO TEXT STUDY QUESTIONS

Chapter 35—Marketing (p. 650)

1. **Do nurses have a marketing orientation? Why or why not?**

   A marketing orientation involves directing your energy towards the identification of the needs and wants of customers and the delivery of services that result in satisfaction. While nurses have always directed their energies toward client-centered care, they have not consistently demonstrated the five attributes of a marketing orientation: a customer-oriented philosophy, an integrated marketing organization, adequate marketing information, strategic orientation, and operational efficiency. This absence may be related to the difficulty with recognizing nursing practice as a business involving services and products.

2. **What is the product of nursing? Of health care?**

   The product of professional nursing practice is problem resolution and quality care provision for clients. Nurses use their knowledge, expertise, and skill to identify problems, implement strategies, and coordinate services to enhance client outcomes. Although intangible, health is the desired product of the health care industry.

3. **How can nurses identify market opportunities?**

   Nurse can identify marketing opportunities by identifying and fulfilling needs (responsive marketing), by recognizing an emerging or latent need (anticipative marketing), or by introducing a new product or service (need-shaping marketing). The identification of marketing opportunities in specific areas of need or interest provides nurses with proactive growth potential.

4. **What is the importance of value and positioning for nurses?**

   Identifying the total value of a product or service and promoting its value position are essential components of the marketing process. As nurses begin to identify, differentiate and articulate the value and benefits associated with nursing service, they will be able to solidify their position as a notable business partner. The establishment of this partnership will be imperative to meet the increasing demands of consumers and health care organizations for the delivery of value-based services.

5. **What is nursing's role in designing the marketing mix?**

   The marketing mix is an individualized blend of marketing strategies used to achieve goals. These strategies may include price, product, and place, or customer value, cost, and convenience, and communication. Nurses can play a role in designing the marketing mix by lowering costs through judicious use of resources (price), delivering quality nursing service (product), within the context of health care arena. As nurses communicate to consumers their ability to provide care that is cost effective, compassionate, competent, and convenient, they will be able to assume a proactive role in the development of the marketing mix.

6. **What image of nursing is held by important target groups?**

   Clients, physicians, and health care organizations are important target groups for nurses. Each target group may hold its own image of the nursing profession; however, the image of nursing is undergoing a metamorphosis. The expanded roles for nurses have contributed to this transformation. An increased number of nurses are being recognized for their knowledge, expertise, and contribution to the health care system. As nurses assume expanded roles such as advanced practice and case management, the image of nurses has been elevated from a subservient one to an image that reflects an autonomous, credible health care provider.

Health Policy and the Nurse

STUDY FOCUS

All countries are faced with the problem of health care needs and the burden of allocating the resources to provide services. A major issue in the United States is whether everyone is entitled to affordable basic health care. An unresolved issue is whether health care is a citizen's right.

Political, social, and economic changes in the United States are creating major changes in health care delivery systems. Nurses must clearly articulate what nursing is, what services they provide, and at what costs in order to compete in a competitive health care environment. Changes in reimbursement methods, increasing demands for services by consumers, and the competition for market share demand that nurses provide accessible, quality services at reasonable costs. Nursing leadership must be active in legislation for health care providers and services. They must also impact policy on reimbursement for nursing services and clearly articulate nursing's role in health care delivery. Nurses must be involved in setting policy.

Policy is the development of value statements, and setting goals and direction. Nurses must also be involved in politics which involves influencing the allocation of scarce resources by setting health policy. *Health policy* is the set of public policies that pertain to health and illness. Health policy can be classified as allocative, which means it subsidizes a group, or regulatory, which means it ensures that objectives are met. The policymaking process is influenced by values. The dominant values in the United States are individuality and competition, whereas nursing values include caring, collaboration, and collectivity. Hanley (1998) proposed a five-step policy analysis framework. The five steps include defining the problem, identifying policy alternatives, projecting consequences for each option, specifying criteria to evaluate each option, and recommending the optimal solution. One strategy that aids decision makers in determining how much health improvement can be achieved per dollar invested is cost effectiveness analysis (Allred et al., 1998).

Public policy is formulated through governmental activities. The policymaking process occurs in three phases and is generally initiated by a small but powerful group, by a widespread problem that affects a large group, or by the media. The first phase is policy formulation, which involves agenda setting and developing legislation. During policy formulation, much debate and input is generated with special interest groups and other influential leaders either to encourage legislation or to prevent a bill. The second phase is policy implementation, which is when the legislation is implemented. At this phase, the law is vague and the details of implementation must be established. The third phase is policy modification. In this phase changes are made as the legislation is being formulated or during implementation. The legislation frequently is modified based on competing viewpoints from multiple constituents.

Legislation at the federal level must go through a multistage process in order to become law. The process has many steps, in any of which the bill can die, be modified, or approved. The first step is to introduce a legislative proposal, also called a bill. Anyone can have input into the drafting of the bill, but only a member of Congress can sponsor the legislation. The member of Congress who is sponsoring the bill introduces it to his or her chamber where the bill will be numbered and referred to a standing committee. Hearings are then held, and the bill is marked up. The committee reports back to the chamber, and the bill is placed on the legislative agenda and then debated. During this process the bill can stand as is or be amended. The bill will either pass or be defeated. If the bill passes, it goes to the other chamber for a similar process. If both chambers approve the bill, it is sent to the president, who may choose to sign it, veto it (a two-thirds vote of both houses overrides a presidential veto), or hold it (it will become law within ten days).

Nurses must be politically active to have an impact on their own opportunities and on client welfare in health policy. Activities that nurses can pursue include calling their legislators, writing letters clearly articulating their expectations and positions, and joining professional organizations to ensure a collective, united voice. Supporting local and state activities, assisting during a campaign for a state representative, voting, and rallying others to vote, forming and participating in a protest rally, and helping draft legislation are other useful activities to influence the legislative process.

Other essential activities include assisting in writing professional position papers through the American Nurses' Association and conducting and sharing essential nursing research studies with legislators who support key issues. Nurses can stay abreast of current legislative activities by reading the newsletters of professional organizations and professional journals, reading newspapers, watching news on the television, and networking with colleagues. Major changes are occurring in health care. Nurses must be instrumental in formulating legislation to ensure nursing's position in the health care delivery system.

Nurses comprise the largest group of health care providers in the United States. The size of the profession creates the opportunity for significant influence in public health policy. Examples of two public policy issues that are important to consumers include the protection of client welfare in managed care and privacy issues in health information disclosure.

LEARNING TOOLS

Self-Assessment

Purpose: To become aware of the strategies for nurses to become politically active in improving health policy.

Introduction: There are many activities that you can engage in to become politically active and support a specific health policy. One strategy is to call your legislators and discuss the importance of a bill or issue. You can provide specific details about why it is important and how it will benefit the public. For example, if the issue is providing reimbursement for nurse practitioners, essential points to discuss are the importance of eliminating financial barriers and improving access to care for families in your state. You can also provide references from nursing research articles about the increased quality, access, and decreased costs for care provided by nurse practitioners to support your position. Additional strategies to support nurse practitioners are referring clients to them, personally seeking care from them, and talking to the community about the important role nurse practitioners play in the health care delivery system.

Follow-up with the legislator by providing a written letter addressing specific points, support for laws on the reimbursement of nurse practitioners and reasons why this is important. Include any resources that might help support your case for expanded reimbursement for nurse practitioners.

Directions: Identify an issue that you are concerned about and would like to see changed or supported by your legislator. Call the legislator, and discuss the issue with him or her. Then send a follow-up letter detailing your position, and include any documents of support. You will find a letter provided, showing you the components to include in the letter to your legislator. It is important to send a typed letter.

Date

Name
Title
Address

To: Name

In this section clearly identify what you expect of the legislator. Example: I would like you to support legislation and policies to remove barriers to equitable reimbursement for nurses in (identify your state).

Describe why it is important for your legislator to support your issue. Example: A nurse practitioner is a registered nurse who has successfully completed a graduate program in a nursing specialty and functions in an expanded practice role. These nurses are able to provide primary care to communities, increasing accessible, affordable, quality health care.

At this point, it is useful to cite statistics or research about the cost, quality, or outcomes nurse practitioners are able to provide. Example: I have enclosed two studies that demonstrate the benefits for the clients of nurse practitioners who provide care. These studies show that the cost of care to clients is decreased, risk factors are identified, and lifestyle modifications are implemented to improve health outcomes.

In this section summarize your request, restate what you expect, and close the letter. Example: I look forward to your support for equitable reimbursement for nurses in (state). Nurse practitioners increase access to care and provide high-quality, holistic health care at a reasonable cost.

Sincerely,

Name, Credentials

CASE STUDY

Jason is an RN on a 45-bed obstetric unit in a large teaching hospital in Birmingham, Alabama. Jason is a primary nurse for both mothers and infants. He always completes a nursing care assessment and then follows up by making a telephone call to track the client's progress. Jason has a population of clients who are indigent and frequently request additional teaching on parent/child care activities. Jason is concerned that the mothers do not have the support or information available to them to provide the best possible care for their infants. Jason conducted a research study on a subset of his clients and divided the group into two. One group received home visits and assistance with nutritional needs, and the other only received a follow-up questionnaire and a single visit to evaluate the parent/child interaction. Jason noticed a marked improvement in the infants in the first group. The infants were more responsive, were more advanced in their activity level, and were all within normal limits for weight gain. The infants in the other group, however, were less active, less responsive, and 30% were underweight for their age. Jason decides that he needs to find a way to support mothers who needs assistance. He becomes politically active to garner support for his interventions.

Case Study Questions

1. What should Jason do to garner support for his ideas?
2. How can his research assist to support his ideas?
3. How long a process is it to change or implement a new program with state or federal moneys?

LEARNING RESOURCES

Discussion Questions

1. What changes in the delivery of health care to clients have occurred as a result of the national health care reform initiatives in the United States?

2. What can nurses do to become politically active and have a strong voice in health care policy?
3. In what phases of the policymaking process can nurses initiate changes to improve the public's health?
4. Does nursing have a strong special interest group in Washington?
5. Describe the multistage process of how a bill becomes law and identify strategies nurses can use to initiate or enhance legislation.
6. What are two public health issues that are important to consumers? Why are these issues important to consumers?

Study Questions

True or False: Circle the correct answer.

T F 1. The three phases of policymaking are policy formulation, policy implementation, and policy modification.

T F 2. Policy issues are raised only when they impact the small, but powerful, groups in the United States.

T F 3. Policymaking is a very analytical process based solely on objective data.

T F 4. Nursing research should be an important component of the policymaking process.

T F 5. Politics is the same thing as power.

T F 6. An allocative health policy ensures that objectives are met.

T F 7. Ethical decisions should remain separate and not be discussed when public policy is set.

T F 8. A white paper is usually drafted by a professional organization to clearly define its position on a specific topic.

T F 9. Politics is the attempt to influence the allocation of scarce resources.

T F 10. The terms *public policy* and *health policy* can be used interchangeably.

SUPPLEMENTAL READINGS

Coopers & Lybrand. (1994). Healthcare reform: Innovations at the state level. *Nursing Management, 25(4)*, 30-35, 38-40, 42.

Johnson, S. (1994). GME financing: A well-kept secret. *Nursing Management, 25(4)*, 43-46.

ANSWERS TO TEXT STUDY QUESTIONS

Chapter 36—Health Policy and the Nurse (p. 667)

1. **What are nursing's major health care values?**

The nursing profession subscribes to numerous health care values, including caring, collaboration, and collectivity. Client advocacy and accessibility to health care are hallmarks of professional nursing values, standards, and practice.

2. **What role do consumers play?**

Historically, consumers have not been active participants in decisions related to health care legislation and politics. As consumers become more knowledgeable, lack adequate health care coverage, and experience spiraling health care costs, their influential role in health care decision has escalated. Consumers are demanding health care reform, improved health care benefits, and a political voice in policy formation.

3. **Is caring a health care policy? Why or why not?**

Caring is an influential element in the formulation of health care policy. While it is not legally mandated, it is a powerful factor in the legislation of policies that govern the distribution of health care resources. Professional nurses bring caring to the legislative arena through political activism and client advocacy for accessible, equitable, and affordable health care.

4. **What kind of public policies govern your life? Govern nursing practice?**

Your private life is governed by the judicial system, which includes laws, taxes, and ordinances. Licensure, practice standards, and each state's Nurse Practice Act regulate your professional nursing practice. Organizational policies, procedures, and protocols also influence the practice of professional nursing practice. Accreditation standards and infection control guidelines, as well as national and international health initiatives have an effect on the delivery of nursing services.

5. **What level of government is responsible for the health of the citizens?**

All levels of government (legislative, judicial, and executive) have a responsibility for the health of citizens. The legislative branch creates bills to enact laws that affect health care. The judicial level oversees civil and criminal cases that influence the direction of health care, while the executive level participates in policy development and enactment, such as Medicaid/Medicare programs and health care reform.

6. **Should illegal aliens be included in health care policies and benefits?**

The issue of health care benefits for illegal aliens is an ethical and financial dilemma. One position espouses that illegal aliens should not be included in health care policy or be entitled to health care benefits. Those who believe that because health care services are financially supported by taxpayer dollars, illegal aliens should be exempt from receiving health care. This sentiment holds true for those who are cognizant of the scarce resources available to meet the needs of the nation's citizenry, as well as legal aliens. Still, some argue that heath is a universal benefit that transcends legality and citizenship.

7. **Why are nursing's professional issues important enough to be on the public policy agenda? Which ones are?**

Nurses introduce policy on public health issues that advocate for the welfare of society. Nursing has been a strong proponent for universal access for all citizens, long-term care, and client rights. Current issues related to professional nursing practice include scope of practice, prescriptive authority, reimbursement for advanced practice roles, and multistate licensure.

8. **Why are politics useful to nurses? What strategies are most successful?**

Politics is a useful tool for nurses to employ as they strive toward fulfillment of professional and personal goals. Politics may be used to influence the allocation of scarce resources, implement change, and develop care delivery systems that enhance accessibility and availability of services. Nurses may select a cadre of political strategies such as voting, campaigning, community activism, and protests to influence public health policy.

9. **Why can nurses be influential in policy and politics? How does this happen?**

Nurses possess the knowledge and political skill to affect public policy. Inasmuch as nursing is the largest group of health care providers, their collective voice can be used to shape policy and politics. Nurses can lobby Congress, form political action committees and coalitions, and hold political office to promote political agendas that advance the health of all people.

Career Development

STUDY FOCUS

Nurses enter the profession of nursing for many reasons. Some enter to help people, others for job security, and still others were influenced by a role model. Nurses may view their work as a job or a career. A *job* is a specific position that one fills for a specific amount of pay, whereas a *career* is a personal and professional plan comprised of a series of positions to meet a long-term goal. Career commitment is an individual's motivation and attitude to work in a professional role. Nurses assesses their personal and professional goals in relation to their work, themselves, and family obligations when determining a career trajectory or professional path. Examining adult life stages when assessing an individual's career trajectory assists in understanding choices throughout the life span in relation to developmental growth and task accomplishment. Early in an individual's career, between the ages of 18 and 22, one experiences an exploration phase; between 46 and 53 one balances one's life, and after the age of 70 one does what one is able to. An individual's career choice is influenced by the work, personal and family needs, and roles in one's life.

Individuals who view nursing as a profession need to plan their career and then follow it up with periodic self-analysis to examine their needs and goals. Self-assessments are important at annual intervals in order to see progress toward personal and professional goals and again at times of decision when choices must be made about changing positions, returning for advanced education, taking a certification exam, or moving to a new location.

Career anchors are personal needs and skills that help to explain individual values in career choices. Friss (1989) identified eight career anchors: service, managerial competence, autonomy, technical-functional competence, security, identity, variety, and creativity. Nurses tend to especially value the three primary anchors of technical-functional competence, security, and identity. An advantage for individuals pursuing a nursing career is the variety of roles available and the multiple part-time opportunities for employment. Many nurses are keenly aware of the social, political, and economic environment that has an impact on opportunities within the profession of nursing, as well as the timing of personal and family goals and demands.

Career planning is essential to meeting professional goals. Career planning is most effective when started early in an individual's career. Self-assessment is the cornerstone of career planning, and finding a supportive mentor is useful to advance your career. Vogel (1990) identified career planning as a lifelong process linked to each person's values, lifestyles, goals, and workstyle. Vogel (1990) identified six stages of career development, including self-analysis, career analysis, integrating, planning, implementing, and evaluating. A written plan is beneficial in formulating your personal and professional goals and your plan should be re-evaluated annually. To meet your professional goals, you must be aware of environmental changes, set goals, plan activities to enhance your career, and anticipate future trends in order to attain additional education or certification. Then you can capitalize on the changing health care environment. Methods for staying informed of health care changes include reading professional journals, reading about current events in the national news, joining the American Nurses' Association, networking, and helping with political campaigns.

Benner's (1982) work describes five levels of proficiency that a nurse progresses through to mastery of content and skill. The five levels are novice, advanced beginner, competent, proficient, and expert. Experience and competence are gained over time and require practice and education. Individuals adjust to the work environment and personal and professional demands while gaining expertise. New graduates are commonly in the novice stage of proficiency, and during the transition from school to work, frequently experience reality shock. Reality shock is when a new nurse faces the challenge of implementing the ideal within a constrained work environment. During this period she/he may become disenchanted. Kramer (1974) identifies the honeymoon, shock, recovery, and resolution of conflict as phases of reality shock.

The health care environment is turbulent and constantly changing. Nurses who strive for a competitive advantage in career advancement may look to future trends to position themselves to capitalize on opportunities. The staff of Nursing 98 prepared 10 predictions about the future of nursing in the upcoming era. Their projections included the following: demonstrating transcultural competence; key role of case management, quality, and customer service as drivers; universal nursing identification system; increased educational requirements; fewer nursing organizations; nurses skilled as data managers; importance of caring and human touch; use of technology to reduce medication errors; and the improvement in language and documentation systems.

Nurses who choose a career trajectory must be their own advocate for advancement and identify learning opportunities essential for their chosen career path. Marketing yourself is important. Finding a mentor, networking, developing and then assessing your career trajectory, and embarking on advanced preparation, certifications, or specialized training may all be necessary to accomplish your goals. Opportunities in health care continually change and keeping abreast of the trends will assist you with career planning. Labor projections and media reports nursing as one of the top ten occupations for job growth. Opportunities are emerging in the areas of primary care and advanced nursing practice. Certification in advanced practice provides recognition by the public of a nurse's specialized area of practice. Advanced education and certification are two methods for nurses to demonstrate competence and quality.

LEARNING TOOLS

Self-Assessment

Purpose: To assist you in developing a career trajectory, and to develop a cover letter and resume to market your special skills and abilities.

Career Trajectory

Introduction: To successfully plan a career, you need to take time to assess your personal and professional goals in order to develop a meaningful, efficient, and rewarding career trajectory. Once you identify your specific goals, you will be able to determine which resources, education, and experience are essential for you to meet your career goals.

Directions: Conduct a self-assessment of your personal and professional goals. Determine timelines for when you would like certain goals met. You may choose to look at early, middle, and late career and lifetime goal intervals. Below, a few categories are listed in which you might identify goals. List those goals that you would like to complete in each time period. Form your goals, then fill in the resource category with what you must do to attain your desired goal. For example, if your goal is to be a nurse practitioner, you must pursue advanced education and that would be put into the resource column.

	Early	Middle	Late	Resources
Career Goals				
Lifestyle Goals				
(Personal/Family)				
Financial Goals				
(Living & Retirement)				

Summary: Complete a self-assessment annually to determine the goals that have been met and what activities you need to engage to accomplish the remaining goals.

Cover Letter

Directions: It is important to write a professional cover letter when applying for a position. Even if you choose to deliver the letter and resume in person, it provides a snapshot of how you present yourself and leaves a strong impression with the recruiter and interview committee. The letter should be clearly written, typed on bond paper, and grammatically correct. Below, a sample cover letter is provided for your review. Take the time to develop your own cover letter based on the position(s) you are interested in obtaining. Make sure you get the correct title and spelling of the recruiter's name.

3195 Hanna Ave.
Detroit, MI 68941

January 21, 2000

Phyllis Jones, RN, MSN
Nurse Recruiter
Cedarville Hospital
719 South Haven
Detroit, MI 68941

Dear Mrs. Jones:

I would like to apply for a position in the six-month graduate nursing internship program for new graduates at Cedarville Hospital that Miss Jason discussed during her visit to Mercy University. Upon graduation with a baccalaureate nursing degree on April 14, 2000, I will be available to begin employment immediately.

Miss Jason's description of Cedarville Hospital as a comprehensive medical center serving the southwestern Detroit community convinced me that the graduate nursing internship is an ideal learning opportunity. I have completed two clinical internships on the medical and surgical units at Cedarville Hospital and have been impressed by the high-quality care provided by the professional nursing staff. I am interested in joining your professional nursing team.

I am available on Tuesdays and Fridays for an interview. Please let me know if it is convenient for you to meet with me on these days. My telephone number is (313) 687-1519.

I am looking forward to meeting with you and discussing the graduate internship program.

Sincerely,

Sharon Smith

Resume

Directions: It is important to develop a clear, concise, accurate resume to convey your work experience, education, and achievements. It is important to devise a simple, but clear format for your resume. Your resume should be typed, free from spelling and grammatical errors, and printed on high-quality bond paper. Gaps between employment dates need to be explained. A brief description of your employment experience is helpful to highlight key performance areas. A sample resume follows for your review. Take the time to create a resume for yourself. This document highlights and markets your abilities. Take the time to make a sharp, professional, accurate resume. It is important that your resume stands out among the others and captures the recruiter's attention.

Meghan Sjots
220 South Appleville Drive
Hudsonville, MI 49604
(616) 245-7894

Objective:	To work as a staff nurse on a medical-surgical unit.
Education:	BSN, Grand Valley State University, Allendale, Michigan, December 1999.
Experience:	
May 1995–Present	Intern, Spectrum, Grand Rapids, Michigan
	Assisted registered nurses in providing direct client care. Assisted with feeding clients, bathing, taking vital signs, calculating intake and output, positioning, and reporting. Certified in CPR.
May 1997–May 1998	Volunteer, Spectrum Health, Grand Rapids, Michigan
	Coordinated recreation activities for the medical-surgical unit. Transported clients for testing and discharge.
Licensure:	Scheduled to sit for the NCLEX in Grand Rapids, Michigan on January 20, 2000.
Professional Organizations:	Michigan Association of Nursing Students
Honors:	Dean's Honor Roll 1995–1999 Kappa Epsilon, Chapter of Sigma Theta Tau Spectrum Health Volunteer Award
References:	Available upon request.

These references are only provided as a guide of what to submit when you are asked for them.

Julie Brown, RN, BSN
Nurse Manager Medical-Surgical
Spectrum Health
1 Spillwood Avenue
Grand Rapids, Michigan 49580
(616) 791-3456

Mrs. Welch
Volunteer Manager
Spectrum Health
1 Spillwood Avenue
Grand Rapids, Michigan 49580
(616) 791-3467

Keverin James, RN, PhD
Professor of Nursing
Grand Valley State University
1 Campus Drive
Allendale, Michigan 49401
(616) 895-3558

CASE STUDY

Janice will be graduating from Grand Valley State University with her baccalaureate degree in December 1999. Janice will be interviewing for her first professional nursing position. She has taken the time to develop a professional quality cover letter and resume. She has researched the available nursing positions in her community and in the surrounding areas. Janice has applied for several positions because of the tight labor market in her area. She is offered two positions—a community health nursing position where she will be a case manager making home visits and helping to coordinate care for a group of families, and a clinical nurse position on a 45-bed medical-surgical unit.

Case Study Questions

1. How should Janice determine which is the best position for her?
2. How does Janice's career trajectory help her make the best decision for her personal and professional goals?
3. Janice has decided that her long-term goal is to become an advanced practice nurse. What is an advanced practice nurse, and how does this plan fit into her present dilemma of which job she should accept?

LEARNING RESOURCES

Discussion Questions

1. How do adult developmental stages relate to career plans and goals?
2. What is advanced practice nursing and how does it relate to nursing careers and career planning?
3. How do health care reform issues affect nursing care planning?
4. What are the stages of career planning?
5. What are the benefits of career planning?

Study Questions

True or False: Circle the correct answer.

T F 1. The most important factor to consider when evaluating job possibilities is the financial remuneration and benefits offered.

T F 2. Career trajectories provide direction as to what resources, experience, and education are needed.

T F 3. The career anchors of managerial competence, service, and identity are most representative of nursing.

T F 4. It is important to stay abreast of changing trends in health care as new options may become available in nursing practice.

T F 5. Career planning is a quick, easy-to-do process that requires little time, but has a big payoff.

T F 6. Advanced practice nursing refers only to nurse practitioners who are in independent practices in rural areas.

T F 7. Career plans or trajectories must take into consideration personal, family, and work-related needs for a successful outcome.

T F 8. A nurse's proficiency level begins with novice and progresses through proficiency, advanced beginner, expert, and then to competence.

T F 9. Midcareer factors include promotions, job changes, and family and personal obligations.

T F 10. Nurses should always be aware of their professional image and market themselves as a career development strategy.

T F 11. Advanced education and certification are two methods to demonstrate competence and quality.

T F 12. In Kramer's phases of reality shock, the *shock phase* is characterized by a time when the nurse begins to learn to cope with the conflict in values.

SUPPLEMENTAL READINGS

Benner, P. (1982). From novice to expert. *American Journal of Nursing, 82(3)*, 402-407.

Greig, B.A. (1999). Career development for nurses in today's health care environment and the value of nontraditional roles. *Nursing Administration, 23(4)*, 63-75.

Kramer, M. (1974). *Reality Shock: Why Nurses Leave Nursing*. St. Louis: Mosby.

Manthey, M. (1999). Financial management for entrepreneurs. *Nursing Administration Quarterly, 23(4)*, 81-86.

Saver, C. (1999). Make the Internet your new career partner. *Imprint, 46(3)*, 60.

Williams, L. (1999). Starting your career. *Nursing Standard, 13(35)*, 59.

ANSWERS TO TEXT STUDY QUESTIONS

Chapter 37—Career Development (p. 684)

1. **Why should nurses plan a career? Why not just follow the available jobs?**

   Nurses should plan a career in order to achieve their professional and personal goals. A career is systematic, deliberate, and sequential process that involves a critical analysis of one's professional, personal, and educational endeavors. Planning a career is indicative of commitment, investment, and active involvement in the profession. In contrast, a job is a fragmented event, used to meet basic security needs.

2. **Why are you motivated for a job or career in nursing?**

   Examining your goals, strengths, and needs will assist in identifying your motivation for a career in nursing. Furthermore, your motivations will be instrumental in the exploring opportunities available in nursing, developing of your career goals, and establishing a career trajectory.

3. **At what developmental stage are you? How does that affect your career planning?**

   Individuals experience the dynamic process of growth and development as they continue through the lifespan. As adults progress through developmental stages, changes that are encountered often impact the balance between work, self, family needs, and roles. Adaptation or adjustment to these changes has an inevitable impact on career needs and decisions. Identification of your current developmental stage through periodical self-analysis will enhance your career development.

4. **How much should your employer contribute to your career development?**

   Regulatory organizations and the community-at-large expect the delivery of competent, quality health care. In order to fulfill this expectation, professional preparation, continuing education, and/or self-directed learning must take place to remain current in professional practice. Employers and employees should collaborate to establish mechanisms that will meet employees' professional growth needs. In order to fulfill the employer's obligation to hire and maintain competent practitioners, the employer should support career counseling and professional development through educational and fiscal contributions.

5. **Is career planning encouraged in your employment setting? Why or why not?**

   Think about your current employment setting. Are mechanisms in place to support career planning and advancement? Is tuition or financial reimbursement available for educational or continuing education programs? Do managers assist you in developing professional goals? Is environment scanning and networking at professional meetings and activities encouraged and supported? Have monies been allocated for such activities?

6. **Why do nurses pursue nurse practitioner certification or licensure?**

   Nurses pursue advanced nursing education, certification, and/or licensure as strategies for career development, professional recognition, and to fulfill state board of nursing practice requirements. The demand for nurse clinicians practicing in advanced nursing roles with greater autonomy is increasing. As health care shifts from tertiary to primary care, advanced practice nurses will assume broader health care roles. Certification is a credential that can be used to assure the public that practitioners have the necessary qualifications to provide specialized services to consumers.

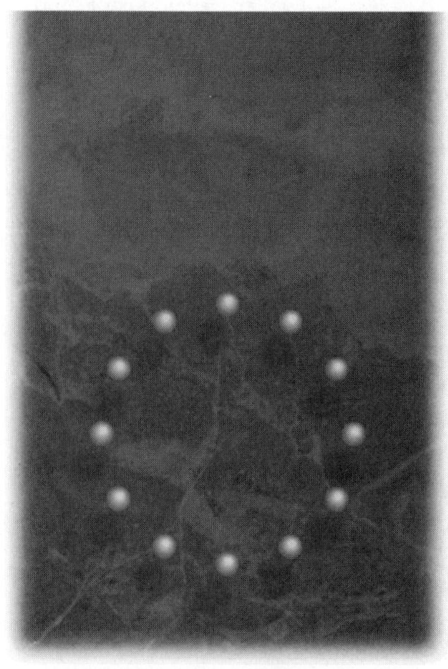

Answer Key

Chapter 1: Overview of Nursing Administration

True or False

1. T
2. T
3. F
4. T
5. F
6. F
7. F
8. T
9. F
10. F

Chapter 2: The Health Care System

Matching

1. D
2. E
3. B
4. C
5. F
6. A
7. G

True or False

1. T
2. F
3. T
4. F
5. T

Chapter 3: Professional Nursing Practice

Matching

1. G
2. A
3. F
4. H
5. B
6. E
7. C
8. D

True or False

1. T
2. T

Chapter 4: Leadership Principles

Fill in the Blank

1. autocratic – direct leadership is needed
2. democratic – direction is needed through facilitation and coordination
3. democratic of laissez-faire approach – to provide direction, but allow group leadership and facilitate team work.

True or False

1. T
2. F
3. F
4. T
5. T
6. F
7. F
8. T
9. F
10. T

Chapter 5: Management Principles

True or False

1. F
2. F
3. T
4. T
5. F
6. T
7. F
8. T

9. F
10. T

Chapter 6: Cultural Diversity

True or False

1. T
2. T
3. T
4. F
5. F
6. T

Matching

1. D
2. A
3. C
4. B

Chapter 7: Legal and Ethical Issues

True or False

1. F
2. T
3. F
4. F

Matching

1. B
2. E
3. C
4. A
5. D
6. F

Chapter 8: Time and Stress

Matching

1. J
2. I
3. G
4. F
5. C
6. D
7. H
8. B
9. A
10. E

Chapter 9: Motivation

Matching

1. G
2. H
3. I
4. D
5. A
6. J
7. B
8. C
9. F
10. E

True or False

1. F
2. T
3. T
4. F
5. F

Chapter 10: Power and Conflict

Matching

1. D
2. C
3. J
4. H
5. I
6. A
7. B
8. E
9. G
10. F

True or False

1. F
2. T
3. F
4. F
5. T
6. T
7. T
8. F
9. T
10. F

Chapter 11: Communication, Persuasion, and Negotiation

True or False

1. F
2. F
3. F
4. F
5. F
6. F
7. F
8. T
9. T
10. T

Matching

1. I
2. J
3. F
4. E
5. H
6. A
7. B
8. G
9. C
10. D

Chapter 12: Delegation

Matching

1. J
2. I
3. H
4. G
5. F
6. B
7. D
8. E
9. C
10. A

True or False

1. T

2. F
3. F
4. T

Chapter 13: Team Building

True or False

1. T
2. F
3. F
4. F
5. T
6. F
7. T
8. F
9. T
10. F
11. F
12. T
13. F
14. T

Chapter 14: Budgeting

Matching

1. E
2. F
3. G
4. D
5. H
6. I
7. J
8. C
9. B
10. A

Chapter 15: Change Management

True or False

1. T
2. T
3. F
4. F
5. F
6. T
7. T
8. T
9. F
10. T

Chapter 16: Staff Selection and Development

Matching

1. D
2. J
3. B
4. E
5. G
6. I
7. H
8. F
9. C
10. A

Chapter 17: Performance Appraisal

Matching

1. I
2. J
3. E
4. A
5. H
6. F
7. B
8. G
9. D
10. C
11. M
12. N
13. K
14. L

Chapter 18: Collective Bargaining

Matching

1. G
2. E
3. F
4. H
5. D
6. I
7. J
8. A
9. C
10. B

Chapter 19: Critical Thinking Skills

Matching

1. G
2. C
3. E
4. F
5. D
6. B
7. A
8. H
9. I

True or False

1. T
2. F
3. F
4. T
5. F

Chapter 20: Decision Making Skills

True or False

1. F
2. T
3. T
4. F
5. T
6. T
7. F
8. F
9. F
10. F

Chapter 21: Financial Management

Matching

1. D
2. C
3. B
4. F
5. E

6. H
7. A
8. G
9. J
10. I

Chapter 22: Outcomes Management

Matching

1. A
2. B
3. C
4. F
5. E
6. D

True or False

1. F
2. F
3. F
4. F

Chapter 23: Productivity and Costing Out Nursing Care

True or False

1. F
2. F
3. F
4. T
5. F
6. F
7. F
8. F
9. T
10. F
11. T
12. F

Chapter 24: Organizational Climate and Culture

Matching

1. B
2. D
3. C
4. D
5. A

True or False

1. T
2. T
3. F
4. F
5. T

Chapter 25: Mission Statements, Policies, and Procedures

True or False

1. T
2. F
3. F
4. T
5. F
6. F
7. F
8. T
9. T
10. T

Chapter 26: Organizational Structure

Matching

1. I
2. C
3. D
4. E
5. F
6. A
7. B
8. J
9. G
10. H
11. S
12. R
13. T
14. Q
15. P
16. O
17. N
18. M
19. L
20. K

Chapter 27: Decentralization and Shared Governance

True or False

1. F
2. F
3. T
4. F
5. F
6. T
7. T
8. T
9. F
10. F

Chapter 28: Models of Care Delivery

Matching

1. J
2. I
3. E
4. D
5. B
6. C
7. F
8. A
9. G
10. H

Chapter 29: Population-Based Care Management

Matching

1. C
2. J
3. D
4. B
5. H
6. F
7. I
8. G
9. E
10. A

Chapter 30: Case Management

Matching

1. D
2. E
3. B
4. C
5. A

True or False

1. T
2. F
3. T
4. T
5. T
6. T
7. F
8. T
9. F
10. F
11. T
12. T
13. F
14. T

Chapter 31: Staffing and Scheduling

True or False

1. F
2. F
3. T
4. T
5. F
6. F
7. T
8. F
9. F
10. T

Chapter 32: Data Management and Informatics

Matching

1. E
2. C
3. A
4. B
5. D
6. F
7. J
8. G
9. H
10. I

Chapter 33: Quality Improvement and Risk Management

True or False

1. F
2. F
3. T
4. F
5. F
6. F
7. F
8. T
9. T
10. F
11. T
12. T

Chapter 34: Strategic Management

True or False

1. F
2. T
3. T
4. T
5. F
6. T
7. F
8. F
9. T
10. T

Chapter 35: Marketing

Matching

1. D
2. I
3. H
4. A
5. F
6. B
7. G
8. E
9. C

True or False

1. T
2. F
3. T
4. F
5. F

Chapter 36: Health Policy and the Nurse

True or False

1. T
2. F
3. F
4. T
5. F
6. F
7. F
8. T
9. T
10. F

Chapter 37: Career Development

True or False

1. F
2. T
3. F
4. T
5. F
6. F
7. T
8. F
9. T
10. T
11. T
12. F